EDOARDO SABATTI

I KNOW YOU TRY

Youcanprint *Self-Publishing*

Title | I know You try
Author | Edoardo Sabatti

ISBN | 978-88-92685-09-3

Youcanprint Self-Publishing
Via Roma, 73 - 73039 Tricase (LE) - Italy
www.youcanprint.it
info@youcanprint.it
Facebook: facebook.com/youcanprint.it
Twitter: twitter.com/youcanprintit

Foreword

"Only those who attempt the absurd will achieve the impossible." (Albert Einstein)

"I know". A very simple statement encapsulates a number of feelings and an amount of power that few others have. Why is knowledge so important? Because knowledge is power. We often underestimate the importance and truth in this sentence, but the author of this book, Edoardo Sabatti, didn't make that mistake. Faced with the arduous task of finding a way to make his son Federico's life better, he attempted what looked absurd, and achieved what seemed impossible.

Lacking the courage to try something new is often what prevents humans from succeeding. Both in the professional and in the personal sphere, the fear of the unbeaten path paralyzes the human mind, or makes it choose the known and safe over the unknown and risky. Edoardo Sabatti understood that he had no choice but to learn and try something he had never seen or considered before, if he wanted his son not to be plagued by severe allergies for the rest of his life. Curiosity -- and maybe a bit of healthy madness, too -- made him discover a cure where he least expected it, in medical equipment that is not widely used in traditional medicine. The device was the answer to most of his questions, and provided some more, making him start a journey into the lives of people affected by allergies (and not only), in order to research and cure their condition.

What is so shocking about Mr. Sabatti's story, that you will be able to read in pages to follow, is its positive outcome for every single person he treated. I am one of them. We tend to think that only in fairytales we can get a happy ending without nefarious consequences, but this book, that documents Mr. Sabatti's life, work and research, will show you the opposite. A treatment that is completely safe, noninvasive and devoid of any medicine or drug whatsoever, can and will drastically improve the health status and quality of life of anyone who is affected by allergies. This book tells the story of a man who didn't accept "learn to live with it" as an answer to his son's condition.

"I know. You… try."

Alessandra Bacchetta

Chapter I

. The storm had just ended, the clouds ran over the mountain summits like the cirrus over the plain of Ireland.

In this village, that bears the austere name of Magno, nothing interesting ever happens. Life runs like a river in the mountains. It follows its ways, already set. Or almost.

Here in particular, people have never moved, not even for love, and the willingness of nothing new has brought generations of blood relationships.

In this submissive mountain village nothing is given anymore, and at the same time nothing is missing.

The privileged position in the valley produces the result that, during Winter, the temperature is four or five degrees higher than in other places, and in the summer, the mountain breeze keeps the heat under the norm, making the area nice and livable.

During the winter season the sun forgets, for two long months, to brush the bottom of the valley. It pokes from behind the mountains and runs fast on the thread line of the slope before disappearing quickly in the valley diagonally, leaving place for the frozen snow and hoarfrost which makes the fencing threads rigid and brightly compact and gives an almost ghostly sense to the contours of the houses and other outdoor things.

This is my village, where I've lived until I got married. It is a hamlet of Gardone in the Trompia valley north of Brescia.

Situated at an altitude of 600 meters, facing east and surrounded by mountains that protect both from the cold north winds and from the summer heat coming west.

Here in Magno, I went to elementary school. I remember that there were only three teachers for five classes.

In January, when I was a boy, I often looked out of the school window. The sky was blue and the fog which covered the valley seemed a white sea of whipped cream.

I was often called to order by the teacher for my abrupt digressions. Strange… I still remember the face and the habits of my old teacher, but I don't remember the name.

In the village there has always been a strong sense of parochialism and although a sizeable portion of the inhabitants of the village works in Gardone, there was always a good clutch of them downtown where here were decidedly different climatic conditions.

Magno had already been recognized as an autonomous village since 1400, in the year of the Lord, while the diocesan recognition as parish came in 1646.

From the soul surviving book, written by a priest and dated 1680, the number of inhabitants was 251, grouped into 40 families of which 10 were Sabatti, like me.

In 1982, Magno was incorporated into the village of Gardone. The old mule track was substituted with the new street in 1950 which was asphalted in 1962.

At Magno in 1968 there were 728 inhabitants of which 166 were Sabatti.

In 2005 I've found through the birth, wedding and confirmation parish registers, together with a meticulous telephone research, the 330 Sabattis in the whole province of Brescia, all of whom descend from 7 original families of Magno.

The families were then reduced to 6 because one family had no heir and was thus unable to pass on the family name. To this family belong the only Sabattis who lived beyond 90 years of age. He was a municipal employee, who died last year at the age of 92.

My family has a higher number of elderly people. The first – born was called like his grandfather. He is 75 years old, is bald and doesn't drink milk since his coming of age. And his son is also bald.

Among them, I have cured the little niece who had a double intolerance to milk and bovine meat, like myself.

One of the Sabatti families instead, counts the oldest member at age 55. So a young family, or rather, a family that does not get old.

The most famous of the Sabattis was Giuseppe Antonio, a civil engineer, born in Gardone in 1757, son of Alexander, renowned surgeon of the epoch and named baron by Napoleon Bonaparte.

The inhabitants of Magno have always shown their great skill as artisans and armourers, specializing in the workmanship of shotguns.

During the Venetian Republic whoever worked in this sector was exonerated from military service.

The balmy climate and a sure job always held my ancestors in their native village.

My paternal grandparents were both Sabatti, even though belonging to two different families from1644.

The maternal grandparents, Tanfoglio and Rizzini, also descended from native families of Magno. And here is the reason for hereditary problems my sister and I have.

My grandfather, my father, my children and I have never met our paternal grandparents. They all died prematurely of illness.

The conclusion is that we 'SABATTI' are a little weak from the genetic point of view.

In the family we were three siblings: my sister Carla born in 1946, myself in 1951 and my brother Bruno in 1959.

My father worked in Gardone V.T. at the Beretta arms factory and my mother, a housewife, rounded off the family budget by doing tailor work, stitching and mending, receiving in exchange farm products such as eggs, meat, cheese, chicken, fruit and vegetables.

My father noticed her in Magno's alleys where she went to visit and sojourn by some relatives during the summer months.

"Who knows what they told each other the first time they met."

He, man of a few words, often taciturn… she certainly was not fascinated by his rough loquacity.

During the Second World War, my mother was drafted into the arms factory where he also worked, my father.

How many things I didn't ask them. How many small and innocent secrets between them I didn't understand.

There wasn't enough time. Time, a not merciful meridian drawn by the gods, to make the humans' struggles aimed at reciprocal knowledge vain.

Of my father I remember the movements, I still feel the familiarity of some of his gestures, that I from time to time during the day unconsciously repeat. And with the help of some old photos preserved in an album I can see his face, but I can't recall his voice anymore.

His voice… that really does not surface from the darkness that wraps my memories.

My father suffered for a long time from different health problems; in 1968 when he was 55 years old he died of a heart attack.

After middle school, I underwent surgery at the right hip for a congenital disease. I was out of school for one year because of plaster casts and rehab for my limb.

At that time my sister entered a convent and became a nun.

The sky is clearing so perhaps God is not angry anymore, I however still am.

Maybe it's not easy for anyone, I for sure can't say that it's all been easy for me.

At that time, there wasn't much public transport for students.

I had to travel four kilometers to go to school from Magno to Gardone, and I certainly was not able to cover that by foot.

So, to go to middle school I went to a college in Chiari which was managed by Salesians. Chiari was a village in the lowland of Brescia that had nothing in common with the village I came from.

The level of cognitive comparison of the school in Magno was far inferior to much the higher education degree that was taught to the pupils of the new institute I went to, and where I was getting ready to learn the first rudiments.

I knew the sacrifice my parents had to make, so I put all my best effort into my studies, and always passed in June.

After middle school, I enrolled in a two year technical-commercial school in Gardone. Meanwhile the bus service for students started working.

After finishing school I couldn't find other employment than some temporary jobs. I even went to the magistrates' court to make some voluntary apprenticeship, being satisfied with obtaining work for no pay.

One year before my father's death I was hired by the Beretta company. The factory usually took in the children of employees who left the job because of pension, accident or death.

I bought a second-hand FIAT 500 and went to an evening bookkeeping course, getting the diploma with great marks.

At Beretta I didn't have a future as a bookkeeper, so I applied for the Economics course at University, whose lessons in those days one could attend after work.

During that year I never missed a lesson. The first exam was math.

For a student who came from an evening bookkeeping course, it was very difficult. But I loved Math and was really interested, so I studied with enthusiasm. 40 students total took the written exam. Only a few more than half was admitted to the oral test.

Only two of the forty participants could solve all the exercises in the written test, one of them was a Sabatti.

The professor turned to me and said: "I certainly can't claim you have copied the written test, considering that the other student who solved all the given questions was on the exact opposite side of the room as you."

I candidly replied: 'In the previous exercises there were some simple traps, in the fifth question it was easier for me to go the opposite way;

that is to say, starting from the final result, I excluded the other three quadrants, I found the first straight line and then reconstructed the other lines in sequence easily."

"But you can't do it that way!"

"You can't start from the roof if you want to build a house", burst out the teacher.

"If you gave me a logical answer I would have given you thirty, but now I cannot give you more than eighteen." replied the professor.

Often, after that day, I found myself starting from the end, to find solutions to various problems of different nature, that life put before me.

Who knows if this personal way of facing certain situations would have disconcerted my old professor after all these years.

The fact is that, since then, I've built quite a few houses.

Following this exam, I passed other hard ones like statistics and law. I also won an open competition as bookkeeper for the hospital in Gardone V.T. The salary was scarce and the job was not satisfactory.

The following year I won another public competition and I was hired by the Bank S. Paolo of Brescia.

I subsequently passed other tests, which allowed me to complete the second academic year.

Working and studying at the same time became, however, more and more difficult.

It took me an hour just to go to work, and then another hour to return home.

At the bank the salary was highly interesting; twice as much, or almost, as that of my jobs until then, so, even if reluctantly, I abandoned my University studies.

To complicate my life, I was also president of a housing association that built cheap council houses in the area near where I lived.

The firm of builders that was building the council houses bankrupted before completing the construction.

The housing association put me in contact with a lawyer, a popular name from a well-known legal firm in Brescia, who already dealt with similar situations.

The lawyer informed me about the procedures to follow in similar circumstances. and without much useless talk, he explained that there were many lawsuits originated by similar circumstances to the one I was examining, but not one had ever been concluded successfully, and least of all were any buildings ever completed.

The only one who could let me complete the work was the bankruptcy trustee with an order from the Court of Brescia.

The Court appointed an estimator, who did not accept any of our observations, and instead limited himself to quantifying the work performed that was not computed.

At the same time, I was careful not to confirm some variations that were asked verbally and that could have compromised my efforts to complete construction work.

In the end I agreed to finalize the payment in two instalments, I contracted the essential jobs at an inferior cost from the previously proposed one in the contract, and with the interest matured on the reserve fund which I managed directly in the bank where I worked, I managed to keep everything within the budget and complete the construction work.

It was my first real success in the strictly operative sphere: since then, others followed, but that doesn't matter, and it certainly doesn't make me any more peaceful and patient.

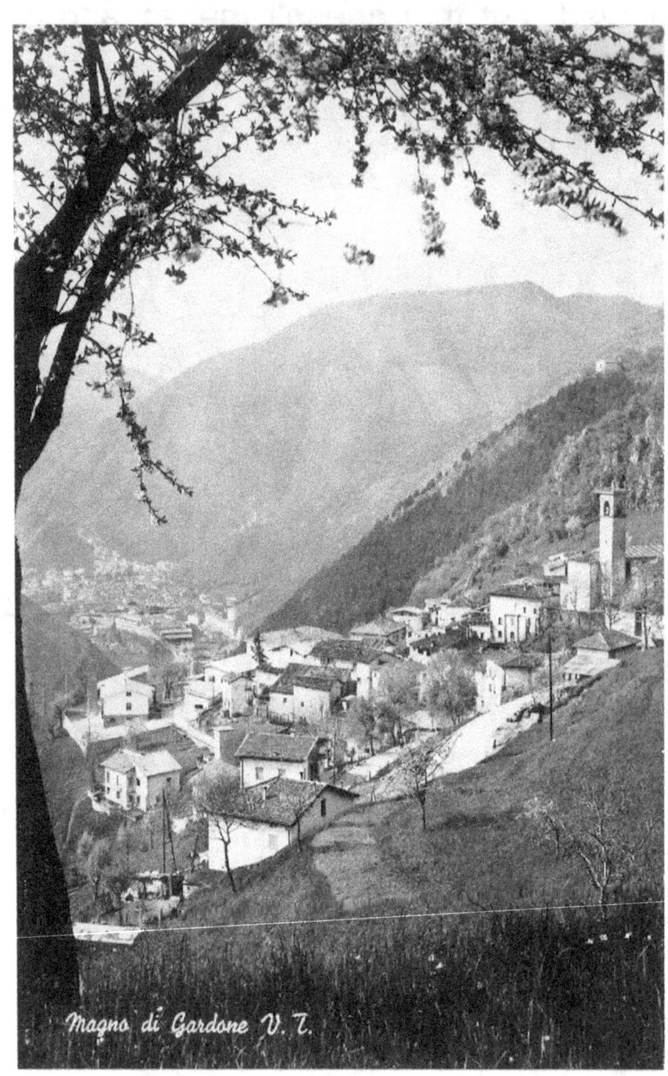

A.d. 1951

Chapter II

17After some time my brother got married, and he restored our parents' house. My mother came to live with me in the new apartment but she did not enjoy this new and unexpected wealth for long: she had a left parietal lobe stroke, and for the remainder of her life, she was completely paralyzed on the right side of her body.

She was in this condition for twenty-four months.

On a day like any other, with the shutters closed, she passed away without clamor, recrimination or pity: she was 66 years old.

A year and a half later I married Mirella.

We moved into an apartment in Sarezzo, still in the Trompia valley, an apt choice, considering that I was closer to my work place and could have more time for personal passions.

As a clever newlywed husband, I decided to take some time to look around in my new village, where I decided to start my next adventure.

In 1990 my first-born Luca was born and subsequently Federico.

Federico was born in July 1993, he was breast-fed for well over 18 months. When he was three years old small red spots started appearing on various parts of his body.

We went for a specialist examination to the pediatric department at Brescia's biggest Hospital, and a well-known doctor recommended that we make another appointment with the head of the dermatological hospital department in Modena, who diagnosed a form of body psoriasis.

That was the start of a series of events that caused consequences and relative choices which would influence me and our events in the coming years.

In October 1996 together with Mirella and my child, I went to the dermatologist, who confirmed that Federico was infected with psoriasis, but he also told us, without so many words, what would be our future.

The psoriasis would progressively deteriorate, year after year and much more so during the winter than during the summer. We couldn't expect miracles or a prompt recovery from thermal water treatments- or from any other kind of medicines.

He also suggested us not to use cortisone products, but to keep them only for emergencies, such as psoriasis patches spreading on the face, because the skin would become desquamate and dry, and that would provoke ulcerous and bloody wounds.

It was therefore important to maintain the skin soft at all times during the day and in every season of the year, and to exploit the only actually effective cures, like going to the seaside, or applying simple economic lotions, with traditionally simple ingredients.

A further suggestion given to us parents was to resign ourselves to live with this problem, and not to put any burden on the child about his chronically deteriorating illness: after all, the child would certainly behave better than us.

In the meantime I continued my work at the bank, and all in all I was doing well there, and I felt perfectly at ease among numbers and financial indexes.

In banking, I could exploit my passion for statistics, applying it to the sector of high finance, to listed stocks, bonds and CCTs and BPT bonds. For bonds, I designed some specific grids, from which anomalous prices would emerge.

The rule was to purchase in lower and to sell in upper.

This was my new world, the horizon gave me a wife, children and a new house.

Sitting on the sea shore, Christopher thought that nothing could end over the columns of Hercules. I, instead, was convinced that my life was all there.

My new world, even if crowned by many successes, was and kept on being flat as the sea without wind.

A lot of people spend their life looking for calm bays and peaceful seas, often without ever finding a safe anchorage. I had all of it at once, but this didn't make me any more satisfied.

Yes, all at once, like in Russian roulette.

When I thought about my mother, her clearest sentence in my mind was: "I don't understand why you asked for a loan for the house, when you had the cash to pay for it."

My answer was always the same one: "For bank employees a very low interest rate is reserved for the first house. fiscally deduct interest and I can invest the loan at a higher rate."

She had always been afraid of debt and had passed her whole life making sure she never got into arrears, even if it was very difficult for her sometimes .This made her heroic in my eyes.

During the first years the bank assigned me to the Stock Exchange department.

There, I met an elegant person who played very hard.

"Lads! Remember that when you play with the Stock Exchange, you can also lose" he repeated to us young people in Brescia dialect.

After a few days I could not help but ask him: "Why do you continuously repeat this sentence and in spite of it you persist in purchasing stock?"

With a smile he answered: "For me, it's like an illness!" In 1960 I had squandered all of my inheritance, but since nobility still accounted for something, I made a good marriage, and in 1973 I also dissipated all of my wife's money.

Now,...I inherited quite a few possessions and cash from an aunt, but I don't know how long they will last."

We were in 1979 and the following year the Stock Exchange crashed, with the tragic recovery of banker Roberto Calvi's corpse.

This encounter made me careful, more prudent with investments towards clients and colleagues that I didn't know very well.

I still have old colleagues who ask for my financial opinion.

Thanks to my banking profession I have had the possibility to get to know people belonging to the most disparate classes and with the weirdest interests.

One day an important customer asked me point blank: "How many shares do you own, from your bank?"

"None" I replied.

"Why?" he asked.

'At the current price I would have sold them all, I'm not stupid" I said.

"So I'm the fool, because your manager has just offered them to me as if it were a privilege!

Now I will go back and thank him." He replied with a wrathful and graceless tone.

I was reprimanded by the bank's branch executive for that financial dispute, to which I replied: "I understand your being reserved, but I don't know how to read your mind. How could I know that you wanted to dump a parcel of shares containing stocks from our bank, exactly at a moment like this and on top of it, that you wanted to dump it on such a wealthy and interesting client for our credit institute? "

Six months later I took the initiative to call that costumer on the phone, and tell him: "the shares of my bank are now down 40% from that famous offer, while bank stocks in general are rising. I think this is a good moment to purchase those shares".

The client bought a good quantity of them, making a good profit within less than three months.

One day, while I was working I noticed him in front of me and without beating around the bush, he asked me: "Would you be my advisor? At the end of the year if there's a profit I'll give you a percentage, but if there's a loss I won't give you anything."

I thanked him for the offer, but I answered: "I am an employee and at the bank I am always at your service, but I don't do anything else."

It was September when a Frenchman came to me.

He wanted to invest in the main shares of the Italian stock exchange.

He often came to the agency to make some bank transfers and I warned him that this was not the best moment to make stock investments.

I recommended him to wait until December 13, Santa Lucia.

This day was propitious for unconditional purchases and statistically less risky.

Besides, it was simpler and more economical to invest in a fund than in single shares.

In the following months the stock-exchange index fell significantly, but he came to me punctually on December.

The safety suitcase he opened in front of my incredulous eyes contained two hundred millions, which considering the risk of such an investment, was a very respectable amount of money.

I invested in different funds and gave him an appointment for May 20 for the sale. On the established date, he came back into my office in order to sell everything, as I had advised.

He had made a 40% gain, and when I left the bank he proposed many different deals, but I had chosen to follow another path.

The company where my wife was a partner needed someone who could take care of the financial side.

At first I asked for a part-time contract at the bank, and that didn't go down too well with the human resources manager, who summoned me and said: "As you are so clever in finance, with the severance pay you will receive, plus the bonus we will give you as part of the package, I suggest you hand in your letter of resignation immediately and devote yourself full time to your new activity."

Times had changed. Working in banking had been a dream for me, but after twenty years the bank was not the same anymore. People had started to speak about budgets, business plans and all those words that were about to introduce the financial world to the speculative bubble of the century, the thing that high finance experts were starting to call "new economy".

Personally I was always interested in new things, but I noticed that most elderly colleagues found it hard to adapt to the changes, and this increased my detachment and decreased my interest for what had been my best career prospect.

It was because of this that I left my work place, even if I had never thought until that moment that I would leave my job at the bank before retirement, and thus even my wife started to tell me:

"If you are so good, why are they paying you to go away?"

In 1999 we built a villa, furnishing it with handcrafted furniture that the charity association my brother works for imported from Peru, and I sold my apartment.

When we moved into the new house Federico, who was six years old confessed to me: "Daddy, when I am big I will never marry, because those who marry, move elsewhere!"

The sky is slowly getting clouded again, I should move and go elsewhere.

Who knows why one must always go elsewhere, and not just when one gets married.

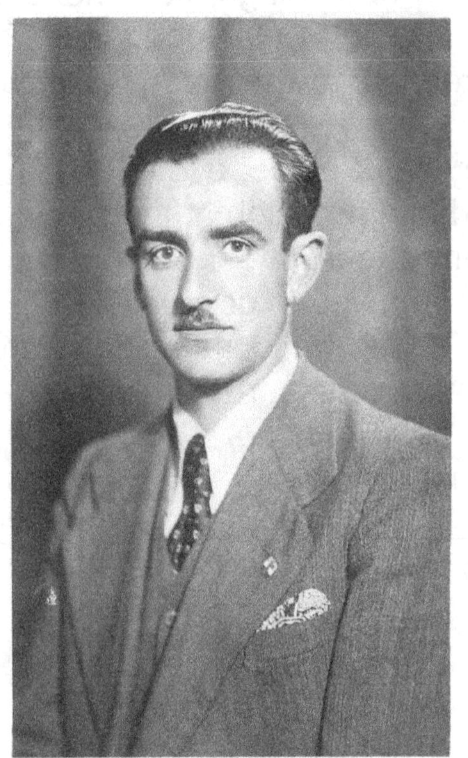

A.d. 1944

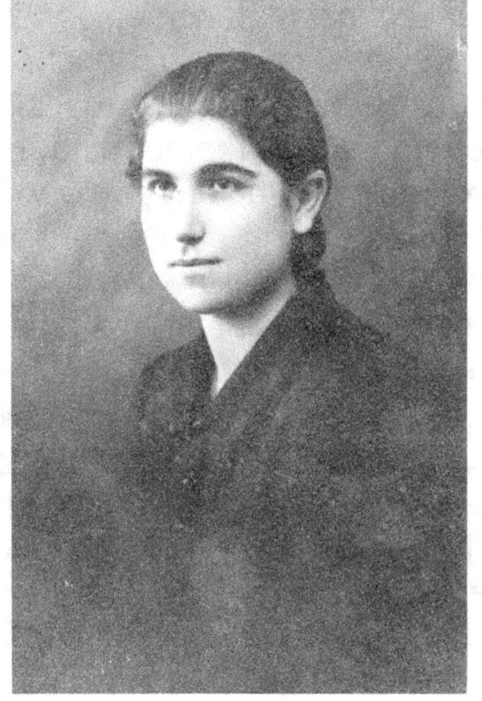

A.d. 1944

Chapter III

In 2000 I suffered a major setback at the stock exchange.

Now if I look back again at my operations I am perfectly aware of the fact that the shares of that year ended their purchasing period with a steep decrease, that also continued into the following years, echoed in 2001 by the collapse of the Twin Towers, with the corresponding drop in indexes and appreciation.

Bonds also suffered some consistent drops. I widened the pattern of my grids, by now all with holes; with continuous daily arbitrages I found myself with longer yield bonds, and higher and higher gains.

So, after a couple of years I started to pay capital-gain tax again.

When the twin towers collapsed the popular saying was that nothing would be the same anymore, an epoch was closing and a social structure was changing which had not been equaled and perhaps would never be again.

Astonished people followed the newscasts. They wandered down roads with a lost look and couldn't believe what was really happening, for how tragic and surreal it was.

Someone said that as of September 11, 2001 nobody would write any more poetry and that no one in love would look at a sunset with the same enthusiasm.

More or less they repeated the same sentences that passed from lip to lip in the years after the holocaust.

And yet, right from the second day after the event, people began to walk and to peek at shop windows, men and women of every age on the third day started to jog in Central Park again, and throughout the streets of Manhattan on day four, Lucy started to walk her dog again. Everything, within a short time, was back to its quiet and sinister normality.

Once I read somewhere that men build sand castles on the beach, the sea hits them with its waves and destroys the work of humans, but men always start over, and build even more imposing castles.

The circle of life is perpetuated again and again and again.

Since 2002 I reorganized the activity of my wife's company, reducing my job to part-time, so I could have more free time for myself, initially devoting the afternoons to my hobbies and subsequently to my research.

In 2006 and in 2008 I underwent hip surgeries. I had to get a prosthesis, with good results.

Now sitting here while I am scrutinizing the sky that delays dusk, I realize that without the support of the bio-resonance these surgeries would undoubtedly have had devastating posthumous effects on my organism.

The bio-resonance has supported my organs giving them the correct energetic equilibrium, it has instructed my cells to a faster and cicatrizing healing process of the wounds, and last but not least, it has quickly cleansed my organism from the congested deposits of the anesthesia.

The electro-magnetic wave resonance: a universe for me then unknown, a cure hidden from my knowledge, and a miraculous source from the cartographic position to me still precluded, and hidden by the too many methodic daily events I had found myself dealing with, in the dark period of my existential knowledge.

Unfortunately for Federico, things went as predicted. In the spring of 1997 the psoriasis had already attacked more parts of the body and the patches of red and ulcerous pustules, sometimes bleeding, were more and more widespread.

As if this were not enough, in the month of July, a form of chickenpox added up to the psoriasis.

This illness had attacked Federico's face, too, making the body and face of the child even more unaesthetic and prurient.

We got wind from friends, that the Thermal baths in Comano in the province of Trento, were specialized in curative baths for skin illnesses.

AlthoughI was skeptical about the existence of such miraculous sources, my wife took Federico to Comano and spent about ten days there.

Federico was visited by various doctors, by the head of the hospital department as well as his assistant while he was there. All agreed in establishing that the illness was running its regular course and that that would then bring on a certain improvement of the pathological conditions.

When he came back from Comano, besides the psoriasis spots, the child also had some small and irritating scabs.

From my part, having noticed the new and unforeseen conditions, I insisted on sending my wife with the child to Comano again for a further specialist examination by the head of the hospital department.

The professor confirmed that the psoriasis had decreased, but as the child was still weak in the meantime he caught another skin illness, impetigo to be precise.

In the professor's opinion this illness was neither dangerous nor contagious but Federico urgently needed treatment for general vitamin restoration.

The child could not attend kindergarten for a long time.

A peculiarity that we noticed during that period, was that every time we were at the sea side Federico's illness receded spontaneously to the point of sometimes going completely away.

In January, thanks to constant treatment together with numerous hospital visits and specific examinations, one enemy was retiring. Only psoriasis was left, to contrast our peace and that of the child.

In March '98 we went together with Mirella and Federico to the island of Mauritius. After a few days, the illness went completely away.

I remember that during the trip back, one of the engines of the airplane failed dangerously. Out of the airplane came a long white trail of fuel.

We remained flying high for over one hour turning round at a height of about 10.000 meters, allowing the captain to discharge 30.000 liters of kerosene into the Indian Ocean. This was to reduce a possible disaster in case of fire during the landing.

My wife and many other passengers said about ten rosaries to the Virgin Mary with fervent ardor, dictated, on top of faith, by an enormous and primitive sense of conservation and survival, while Federico and I, like two unrepentant gambling den members, played cards and exchanged glances with artful understanding.

In May '98 we were called by Federico's kindergarten teacher: "The child is not feeling well, if you could come immediately…"

This was all relayed to us with a calm voice.

When we arrived there, the child's face was already swollen. He had had ham and a kiwi for lunch.

We immediately took him to the ER at the hospital in Brescia, where we discovered an anaphylactic shock caused by his eating kiwi.

This food intolerance of Federico's to kiwi added up to the already burdensome problem of the skin illness, the difference being that we had always to bring with us an antihistamine drug, to avoid the danger of another and more dangerous shock, which according to the doctors could have been fatal.

Thus began a long, incessant and frantic run for allergic tests.

After various skin tests it was verified that Federico had different allergic forms and various intolerances, such as allergies to: pollens, dust, grass, pork, cocoa, milk, eggs, tomato and potato.

Further detailed tests found traces of lead and a massive organic absorption of copper and manganese.

An alarming allergic picture of significant nature, the ideal study area for anybody who recently graduated in spontaneous or induced allergies, or for specialized technicians in environmental technologies and food.

In March '99 I decided to go on a cruise in the Caribbean.

The four of us started with a lot of enthusiasm that was motivated, the holiday was in fact fantastic and in some ways adventurous and sensational, even if for Federico's psoriasis it was not the magic healing we had Hoped for.

For me, on the contrary, this new break from the daily grind was intense and liberating. It was as if this thin sense of anguish and emptiness that was always inside me, had never been allowed to rest.

Now that I think of it, I may never have been as happy as I was at that time.

On January 14th, 2000 while we are having lunch at my in-laws', Grandpa cuts a kiwi, Federico touches the peel and grates it with his nail and afterwards licks his finger with the tip of his tongue.

There is no immediate reaction.

I serenely go to the office that is about 500 meters from my wife's parents' house.

After a while I receive a call from my mother- in- law who, with agitated voice informs me, "Federico has red eyes and his face is swollen".

The race to the hospital of Brescia is frenetic and breathless .When we arrive at the reception of the ER, where they immediately hook him to IV lines, Federico's head is significantly swollen.

When he is discharged, the doctor suggests that we always carry some adrenalin with us, because next time the child could not make it to the hospital.

Ever since, there was no need to tell

Federico to stay away from kiwi at his classmate's birthday parties, at the parochial festivals, at meetings of the youth groups or other gatherings: he didn't eat or drink anything anymore, and above all he stayed away from everything what was green.

Twenty days later we all went to the Sinai peninsula.

Sharm el-Sheik, the highly in demand and advertised holiday place, presented itself in all its uncommon and barbarous splendor.

In the middle of the sea the island of Tiran emerges from the depths of the ocean like a precious and lonely pearl. Behind lies the Exodus desert with its mountain tops that, starting from the mountain of St. Catherine rise up to the mount of God; the rocky desert, with only a few dunes, entombed the patriarch graves, trampled on by prophets and saints, an amphora for the food of the omnipotent.

Federico did not bathe in that crystalline water that offers the vision of one of the most beautiful reef barriers in the world, and he s too timorous to plunge into a decidedly cold sea during that tepid month of February.

On the other hand, much to my amazement, the psoriasis was completely gone after the first week.

Certain places, particularly those where the sea was present, had strange powers on Federico's skin; they could give that relief where incessant treatments could do nothing.

Nature had the capacity to cancel the suffering which she herself had caused, venom and antidote coexisted in the same bosom, even though I still didn't know how to find the solution to this controversial problem.

Unconsciously, only now I realize, I had found my path, yes, my path, because until then I had wandered through the streets of life without any purpose.

I've always believed that each one of us has a road to follow in order to find themselves and God, but I had never thought that I, too, had something to do both for myself and for others. Or rather, I had never done anything to uncover the secrets that life had in store for me as well.

I raise my coat's collar; I clench my shoulders to smother a strange shiver that runs down my back. I look high at the clouds that move towards the mountain tops, the day is finishing its song.

What a strange coincidence, in the distance a passer-by on the road going up the hillside is looking at the sky and he is raising the collar of his raincoat.

Now I'm feeling quieter and perhaps a bit less alone.

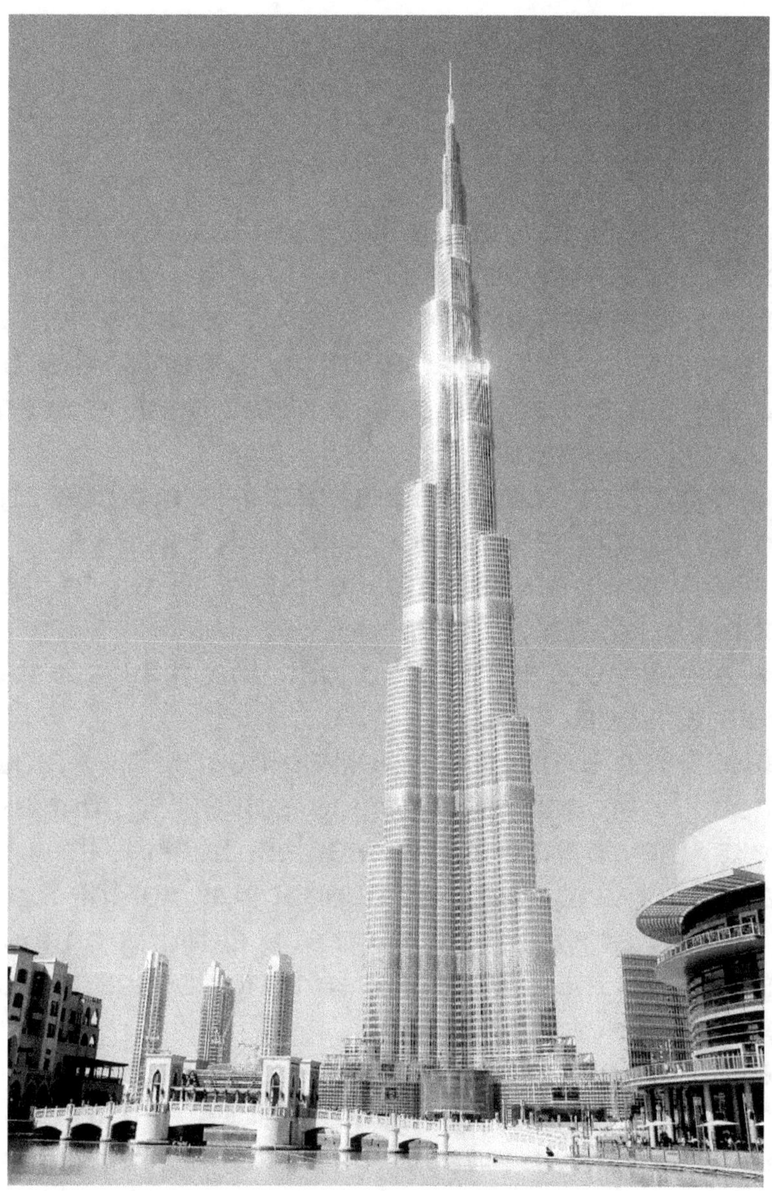

Dubai 2010. Every time men start over, and build even more imposing castles.

Chapter IV

Suddenly, a gust of wind shakes the tree tops.

Unexpectedly, a memory appears clearly in my mind.

I see -- playing like in an old film -- many scenes which are fragmentarily superimposed: the old house of my parents, the bench in the square where my father sat and talked about hunting scenes and real life happenings with his friends.

Life was hard for him, too. The last of three brothers, he had been left an orphan by his mother when he was only three years old.

He fought the war in Africa, and he often talked to me about that dark period of his existence.

The stories always began with hunger, the only constant that was present in every episode.

One day after three exhausting walking hours, they reached the Tana Sea. Somebody thought of catching some fish, but as they didn't have any hooks, they bent sewing needles. Luckily, they found something to use as bait and for that day hunger was not the master.

Another time they arrived exhausted at a clearing on the border with the savannah. While they were assembling the camp, they noticed some monkeys on the nearby trees.

Their strident and deafening noise was disturbing the soldiers.

Suddenly, a soldier, picked up some stones and threw them at the monkeys. The monkeys ran away and for a while there was silence.

Then they heard loud noises again. The monkeys were back in their previous positions, in their natural habitat.

This time they made the soldiers run away by throwing big stones in every direction.

What's certain is that things that can damage others are learnt easily, and just as easily, they can be put into practice.

After the war, the factory group my father worked with often organized trips using trucks. By this means, complete with self-sacrifice and with a lot of enthusiasm, they managed to visit some big cities like Milan, Turin and Florence.

The immense passion for adventure brought them one day as far as Monte Carlo, where all the participants drank a terrible and bitter coffee at the end of the meal, because nobody knew how to say sugar in French.

I've always known that education makes life easier.

Times changed: at six years of age, Federico updated me on the performance of the Nasdaq, that he saw on Bloomberg.

A sudden flashback paints the figure of my father during the summer evenings, while he rolled some national tobacco in worn-out cigarette paper.

On Sunday afternoons, he liked playing "tresette" at the village inn, and drinking a glass wine, rigorously red.

His black and white photo has always been sitting on the cupboard in cherry wood in the corner of the kitchen, from where with its retro look, it seems to study everybody who comes into the house.

It has been there for over 40 years.

When my mother died, I bought a double frame and I placed photos of them both one near the other as it always had been, and as it should have been.

I've always loved the sea, it is my natural environment.

When I was single and a banker, I always asked to take my time off for the summer holidays in July.

Every year I changed destination: Sardinia, Sicily, Elba; my travelling companion was often a friend from my village whose name was Federico.

That summer I was alone and I decided to go to a holiday resort in Calabria.

When I arrive, I put down my luggage and go to dinner; there I hear somebody speaking with a Brescian accent.

A good-looking, distinguished woman, gentle in aspect and quiet in dialogue talks with great enthusiasm about her conquering her first regatta win by herself.

I am dazzled. If a skinny fifty-year-old woman can sail by herself, so can I.

I thus learned that I could take a course to become a master sailor.

I've always thought that one day I would take the rudder of my life in my hands, finally the right opportunity came along.

So that year, I approached the first rudiments of lone sailing.

The following year I went to Numana, south of Mount Conero near Ancona, where I could perfect my previous sailing course, and in addition I could sail with big catamarans, that are very stable because they have two hulls.

That year, I succeeded in various impossible missions. I even overturned with a catamaran, smashing a buoy that was the tip of an iceberg because underneath it, a huge group of mussels was growing.

In September the same year I went to Corfù, and stayed at a holiday resort that was very popular for those who loved sailing.

During the morning I could take a big boat that took us to beaches that could only be reached from the sea, and there I could see all sorts of fish like octopus, moray and many different sponges.

In the afternoon using the same boat, we could make some panoramic excursions in order to look at the

coast. This made me try my hand at steering a real sailing boat complete with crew and passengers, including an irreverent French dame, whose duty was to supervise the maneuvers of the race.

I took over the steering of the rudder with enthusiasm, yes, the nice rudder, the wheel with the knobs outside made of brass, the one you see on pirate ships, just to be clear.

At the beginning I sailed skillfully, paying attention to the big compass, keeping to the foreseen route, but Aeolus was blowing in a different direction and it deflated the white sails, irritating the pink corsair who took the rudder while cursing.

Puffing and panting, the lady gave it back to me commanding: "Helmsman let's veer….. course south-east".

I took some fantastic trips with the sailing boat in coming years, until during a regatta with a girl coming from Milan, a twister that overturned the boat in open sea knocked us down.

We were both luckily saved by an English man who was on a big outboard boat.

With Mirella things were getting serious: we had been speaking about marriage for quite some time, so I knew that the sailing boat had no future.

As if that was a bachelor party, I went to the Maldives, to one of the few resorts that had sailing boats at its disposal.

I therefore arrived on a small Maldivian island with only 20 bungalows.

The island was in an atoll. The water was low, at the extremity there's the reef, the cliffs go vertically down: nice to see for those who loved diving, but not for swimming, the water is cold.

The island staff tells us that it's best to stay still if we are unfortunate enough to meet a shark in the sea.

The thing that impressed me the most were the sea shells, big and arranged like suitcases at the train station, orderly, in line, but without rigor.

When slightly open, they let you peek at the mollusk, that looked like a colored silk foulard designed by a famous stylist.

Super slow angelfish with black, white and yellow stripes, with a long white caudal fin.

Butterfly fish, a couple of fish swimming one in front of the other, yellow with black spots or purple with yellow spots. Pajama Cardinal fish, yellow with black stripes, Parrot fish, very colorful and so called because of the beak that crushes the coral, globefish, crossbow fish and huge hermit crabs.

One day I follow a giant green turtle while it dives, and when I resurface I have a grey shark in front of me.

He is a couple of meters away from me. I see him from the side, his head on the left and his tail on the right. He is much bigger than me.

There sure was no need to tell me to stay still. I was literally paralyzed.

A few centimeters from the surface I was observing this war machine, triangular fins, the left black eye, I see him breathing through the gills then… in the blink of an eye, he turns right, a tail smash and he disappears into the blue ocean.

At long last came the monsoon from north-east, the dry and constant one that allows you to sail inside the atoll. I hear some whistles but I don't see any birds in the clear sky, I hear waves moving and I see some small black dolphins, passing my catamaran.

Where you find dolphins you will not find sharks and whenever for a short while I was not in the good company of these genius mammals, I felt my heartbeat increasing.

I sure heard plenty of bizarre stories, like the one of the pair coming from Venice I knew on the island.

They married the year before, they had booked the same resort that I had chosen for my sailing, a few days before departure, the agency informed them that the flight was cancelled and as a solution they proposed to put them on a flight for Zürich that made a stop at Colombo before reaching the Maldives.

They accepted the change and went to Zürich by train, the Swiss airplane landed in Sri Lanka while there was civil war.

They remained there for 24 hours without getting off the airplane and then they were authorized to return to Switzerland.

After many complaints, announcements in the newspaper and legal actions for a reimbursement for the trip, they are given the chance of travelling with Alitalia, direct flight from Milan, but this time at Milan/Linate there is too much fog and the flight is transferred to Genoa, essentially they arrive at the resort 18 hours later.

Or like the boy from Faience, who went to the Seychelles every year to sell ceramics to the local artisan shops, that the tourists bought as souvenirs for their Italian relatives and friends.

The water clearer than the sky, walking at midday on the coral beach that never burns, getting to know people, the most disparate… all of this produces an unforgettable sensation.

Here, now, I remember everything clearly: this takes that subtle discomfort away from my mind, and the shiver down my shoulders seems to abandon my body.

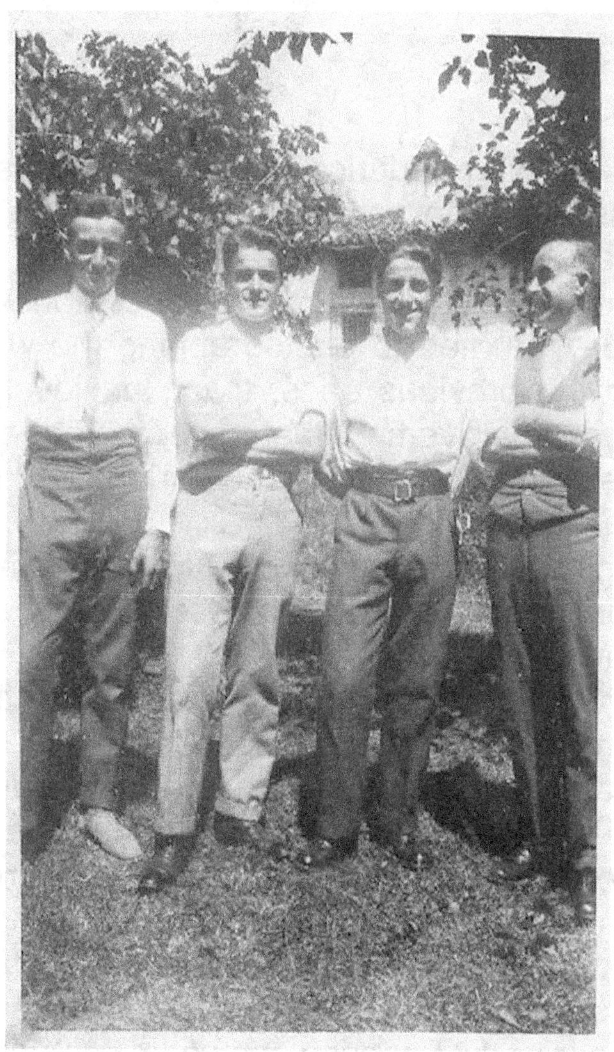

Grandfather Carlo with his three sons A.D. 1935

Chapter V

Every Sunday morning Federico took a bath with salts That cleaned the wounds caused by the psoriasis and when he was dry I photographed the big spots he had on his shinbone.

During the week I used two different products, one for each leg.

Then on Sunday I turned to photographing the wounds and I compared them with the previous ones, trying anxiously to find in these immortal details, an improvement that never happened.

I tried about ten different creams and various ointments without getting significant results.

After three months I stopped taking pictures. It was depressing to see how it deteriorated, but nevertheless I continued using the two creams during the week.

The sand in the hourglass placed on the shelf of the fireplace in my study, had slid many times from top to bottom.

I had done that for a long time , it helped me govern events. Every time I was alone in my study and thinking about Federico's situation, it was a spontaneous gesture for me to turn the old time recorder upside down; it gave me the impression of having a vague handle on time.

The months passed all the same. In May of that Holy Year, my nephew prepared himself to receive the sacrament of Confirmation.

During the dinner party, Federico showed clear signs of distress.

It was the day when his favorite football team played the last game of the Serie A championship in Perugia.

After saying goodbye to the guests, Federico went over to his grandfather and said: "Today we "Juventini" (Juventus supporters) have an appointment with history; after that we can come back".

The hard-fought match was suspended because of rain, while rival team Lazio won.

Federico started to become worried about the final result, silently at first, and then more and more loudly.

"With this field we risk to lose. How can I ever show myself in front of my friends again and more importantly in front of grandpa?"

It was late, and returning to the dinner party was no longer possible.

It was his grandfather who instead came to our home, while Federico looked strained and very preoccupied playing "table football".

Grandpa spoke to him in a sneering tone and asked : "What did Juve do?"

Without rising his head Federico answered: "they lost, but… it's not important!"

When his grandpa said "What? It isn't important after you've spent a whole year talking to me about nothing but football?",

Federico stopped playing and looked him in the eye: "Grandpa, health is what matters."

Helping Federico had become a sort of obsession; how and where there was remedy I was so desperately seeking, even I still didn't know.

I found -- not without quite some difficulty -- a Spanish silver-based spray that alleviated the psoriasis for a couple of months, but then the illness got back to the previous state.

I started trying all sorts of homeopathic products, pharmaceutical concoctions suggested by different dermatologists, and I consulted many specialists including an iridologist who prescribed products with a magnesium, copper and zinc base.

This time Federico did get better, with the psoriasis turning a lighter receding for quite a few months.

At that point, I recommended the same doctor to my nephew, who had a light form of psoriasis on his hands, and the iridologist ordered him to use the same products.

Later on, I found out that that another person with a completely different problem from Federico, went to see the iridologist, too, and the doctor prescribed him the same identical products.

An acquaintance spoke to me about another iridologist who was less "mainstream" and more technologically advanced than the first one.

This man photographed the pupil with the help of a small digital camera and immediately obtained a computer image of an enlarged iris having therefore abundant time to study it in detail.

From the monitor, it was clear that Federico was showing traces of evident physical and psychological stress. Signs of stress that were unusual for a boy his age.

As far as the products Federico was using, he suggested to continue with the magnesium, suspend the copper and to absolutely stop using the zinc, as the already ingested quantity would suffice for several years.

He also told me that we could do tests on the hair, different from those we had already carried out for allergies.

An American company from Phoenix needed a quite a relevant quantity of hair, the closer as possible to the root.

This made me curious, so I sent both children to the barber's, I delivered the two samples to the specialist, and within a month I got the answer.

Federico, although constantly taking magnesium, needed a huge quantity of it. His hair also showed traces of nickel and cobalt; as far as toxic metals there was a relevant quantity of aluminum and the ratio between the various metals was completely missing the normal parameters in most cases. Luca's parameters instead, were within normal limits for the most part.

Among dietary suggestions, he told us to reduce carbohydrates, and pasta in particular.

It was the year 2004 and pasta was the only food that the Italian allergy tests didn't reveal as dangerous. I was confused.

During the month of June I had some work problems.

Our church had organized a summer camp in Senigallia in the Marches. The boys were growing up and clearly manifested a preference to spend the summer holidays with kids their own age, rather than with their parents.

I recommended Luca to look after his brother and so we agreed, even if reluctantly, to their request of participating in this adventure, which was a new life experience for them.

After only two days, Luca tells me that things are not going so well. The house where they sleep is one kilometer away from the beach and when they come back at one o'clock in the afternoon it is very hot, they sweat and there are so many of them that they don't manage to shower before lunch.

Federico calls me telling me that his skin on his whole body is burning. He lets it slip that perhaps it is better to put up with his parents and live in a healthier and more comfortable environment.

The following day, Luca as well states that he is worried about the wounds on his brother's back, and expresses a few reserves on the menu, about the types of products used, that are not completely in line with Federico's physiological needs.

We reach a compromise.

On Saturday the first week ends. At 6 a.m. we will drive by, to go to S. Benedetto del Tronto, and we tell the boys clearly that whoever wants to come with us must have their luggage ready.

We arrive at Senigallia at 5.45 a.m. and find the boys Read, luggage in hand.

Federico was doing very badly. He had ulcerous wounds on his torso, arms and legs. Certain parts of his body had the skin burned and rolled up.

He is clearly dehydrated, so as soon as we are at the hotel I make him soak in the bath tub, and I send Mirella to buy three boxes of moisturizing lotion.

Pampered with a lot of treatments and attention, Federico goes back to an apparent normality within a few days.

That same week I meet Franco again at the hotel. He is a psychologist friend who talks to me about a center in Milan where electromagnetic bio-resonance is used to cure various illnesses.

This news makes me very curious, but unfortunately the waiting list at that center in Milan is very long.

I start my research and I hear that in Brescia a general practitioner has bought the same machine. He has shorter waiting times for the first visit, but longer for food tests.

This machine is called BICOM 2000.

The search continues once, back from the holiday, I find a lot of information on the internet in various languages, but not much in Italian at all.

One of these websites says it is a miraculous remedy and talks about excellent results in a very short time.

Starting from this premise, I call the doctor explaining that it is urgent.

During the first meeting the doctor discovers the allergen that causes most of the problems.

He insists on eliminating all products that belong to the category enabling the allergen, and then specifically states that, besides not ingesting foods that provoke intolerance, one must also avoid any skin contact with such foods, as magnetic frequencies can emanate through gloves, glasses and paper wrapping food.

In addition, he also gives us a leaflet containing lists for hundreds of products that are compatible for patients with the same intolerances.

He also suggests us to bake our bread at home, because industrial and artisan ovens cannot guarantee the use of products that don't contain substances that might trigger food intolerance.

At first glance, the testing method of this machine seems extremely simple, almost primitive, so much so as to cause doubts on the machine's real potential.

During the visit, while connected to the machine by an electrode in one hand, you carry out a strength test with the fingers of the other hand: thumb and middle finger closed together, forming a ring shape. The doctor tests if and how the fingers can hold, when he tries to separate them, breaking the ring they form.

Not only the doctor but the patient, too, can notice if there is a reduction of their strength. This indicates that the connected substance is not well received by one's organism.

The test for children, who do not have the capacity to hold their fingers tight forming the ring, is carried out by forming a chain with the parent.

The child holds the electrode in one hand and puts his other hand in their parent's. The doctor takes the test with the parent's hand.

I ask to verify the effect of kiwi, the doctor confirms that the fruit was not good for Federico, but that it wasn't important. He claims that if we treat the allergen correctly, the other intolerances will become less aggressive.

This doesn't convince me. On the contrary, I am quite perplexed.

Following this first visit, I take my brother and my brother-in-law's Family, as well as other good friends to do the test, and this allows me to get more information to answer my questions.

The treatment that the doctor prescribed for us is a strict three-month diet.

Adults must take some detoxifying vials once a week, and afterwards they will be tested with different food products.

I don't want to wait that long.

The tests seem very effective to me, I would like to check foods, soaps and other objects such as watches or cell phones, medicines and much more.

I am sure that the machine can give me many more answers.

The doctor doesn't want to move the machine from his study as he is very busy with his patients and with his research already. So I seriously start thinking about buying this machine.

I begin to research again, and I only find one sales agent in Italy who sells this kind of machine, he is in Milan.

I contact him at the end of July and he offers me the machine compete with accessories and vials for beginners at a cost of 33,000 euros.

After much consideration, I decide to buy it.

I complete the payment. The bio-resonance instrument is called BI-COM 2000, made by REGUMED, a German company.

It will be delivered at the end of August.

Upon delivery, I am entitled to a one-day course to learn the main functions of the machine.

I am also given a volume with directions on how to use the machine and a volume for all the treatments.

Among the accessories there's one called "Birek", a metal wire with a small parabola at one extremity and a heavy handle at the other.

It is a hand instrument and if you place the parabola between your hand and the plate it oscillates: horizontally if the signal is negative, and vertically if the signal is positive.

When it doesn't oscillate and remains still, it is by definition in a neutral phase.

The salesman insists that it is necessary for me to exercise with this instrument, that makes the tests easier and much quicker, compared to using acupuncture on fingers, that is more difficult and more painful for the patient.

From the first test I discover that Federico and I have the same intolerance to milk and beef while Luca and Mirella show intolerance to beef only.

I read and reread the instruction book, the Birek slowly starts to move, I start testing all the products I have at home, I eliminate a type of bread, wine, some types of pasta, some soaps and one shampoo.

I need to create a list of products that cause intolerance for Federico.

I ask and obtain an authorization to check all the products in our local supermarket, that was owned by a relative of my wife.

These tests can only be carried out on Monday when the supermarket is closed.

I manage to confirm the first few things. It is not true that all the wine is not good, but unfortunately the cheapest gives very negative result. The majority of wines sealed with crown or screw caps is negative, while wine in bottles with corks is positive.

Generally speaking with regard to alcohol, the cheapest products also test negative.

Bread works the opposite way. Common bread without additives is positive, while soft bread and toast bread with additives and preservatives, produces very negative results, and not only for those who have a slight intolerance, but for everybody.

The first few animated family discussions took place as a consequence. I certainly couldn't tell my wife that bread was bad, as she came from a family of several generations of bakers.

As we had often had lunch with in-laws, I asked for common bread only to be on the table And I brought the wine.

By eliminating beef and milk completely from Federico's diet, all the psoriasis signs disappeared.

By following this type of dietary restrictions, that the bio resonance suggested, we are all feeling much better.

My constant stomach-ache gradually fades, while in the morning my leg muscles are less and less rigid, that thick white paste on my tongue disappears, and I also start losing weight without giving up too much food.

As is in my character, I start digging everywhere, into everything and in every possible direction; there's a problem to solve, and the solution finally appears to be at hand.

My research moves on to the hereditary characteristic of food intolerance, so I start testing all my relatives.

The most important intolerances are three: milk, meat and eggs.

The percentage of those who are intolerant to these foods among my relatives is 100%: a lot of them have a double intolerance to beef and milk while others only have one intolerance.

At first I start thinking that literally everyone is intolerant to a type of food, until I discover that my dentist has no problem whatsoever with any food, I check his daughters that are like their father, while his wife has one intolerance.

I start testing big families, I find that the parents had several allergies, while the children are for about one half like their father and the other half like their mother.

Younger children have significantly fewer intolerances than the older ones: generally speaking, the younger ones are only intolerant to one type of fruit, as opposed to the four or five types for parents and older siblings.

I find one daughter who is completely different from her parents, later they inform me that they have adopted her.

I test a woman who is older than me, and find the double allergy to milk and beef. I ask her where she lives and where her parents come from, I find out that her name is Sabatti and she lived in Magno when she was a little girl. She remembers my parents, her father was my dad's cousin, she still has an aunt who lives

I test my wife's brother. He has four children and two have the same allergic factor as he does, while the other two are like his wife.

I find out that my wife has the same food intolerance as her mother while her brother is identical to their father.

After gathering a significant amount of data, I notice a constant. Children who have the same food intolerance as their mothers were born at the end of the full cycle of pregnancy, with the mothers enjoying a calm gestation, whereas those who had different intolerances from them, often caused a few problems to the mother during pregnancy and in several cases were born before their mother's due date.

My wife, too, had enjoyed a calm gestation with her first pregnancy. Our first son was born a few days after her due date, whereas with Federico, she was twice hospitalized, and he was born before her due date.

My mother-in-law had experienced no problem while she was pregnant with her daughter, whereas she had a lot of problems with her son's birth.

My brother's wife had experienced many problems with her third child, while my brother-in-law's wife,   while not experiencing any particular problems, delivered the children with a different allergen from hers before her due date.

I tested over two hundred couples but less than 10 per cent had the same allergen, and from the statistic point of view, this is certainly an anomaly.

My grandfather was bald, my father was too. I do not smoke, I stopped drinking milk and coffee when I was 20, and I do have some hair left.

Among my male relatives, all the bald ones have an intolerance for milk and many of them have stopped drinking it when young, because of gastric problems.

My research is confirmed when I test other men: the majority of those who lost all their hair while young, were intolerant to milk. Luca's pediatrician doesn't believe it, but he smokes, he has an intolerance to milk and he is bald.

Chapter VI

There must be a strange gene in my deoxyribonucleic acid that causes tenacity.

Everything I had to face in my life up until today has never daunted me, on the contrary, it has always been like a strange protein charge that spurs me to research, and to find a solution for every question.

I remember a friend who came from abroad with the novelty of the Rubik cube and for a whole week, he had tried to find the solution, but without any success.

He gave it to me around midnight, with a hopeless air to himself.

As soon as I got home I started composing it, the upper surface, the first two crowns, and so on, with pen and paper to count the small squares and then calculate the chances to insert them.

The following morning at 6 a.m. , satisfied like an intelligent being who has discovered fire, I looked at the cube that was lying on the kitchen table with all its colors in the right place.

As long as anything was strange and full of difficulties it was interesting for me and it spurred me on to find the solution.

This was the reason why I took on a subject that was semi-unknown not only to most people, but also to Italian traditional medical and pharmaceutical science.

I therefore enrolled in some peculiar and quite unknown alternative biomedicine courses that taught us how to use and optimize the use of the electromagnetic bio resonance; they also trained us on consulting the machines to perform the bio resonance, as well as using alternative medicine practices, and instructed us on energy studies tied to traditional Chinese medicine.

During the first refresher course, I showed up with a lot of questions and arguments that I had written on my small and super personal diary.

There were over twenty enrolled students, most of whom were doctors.

When the lecturer, an austere German professor, asks how many of us are systematically using the BICOM, only three of us raise our hands, me included.

This helps me overcome my initial awkwardness. I ask my first few questions and I am ridiculed immediately.

The comment of the amused German is immediate: "What, you bought BICOM just to carry out allergy tests?

In order to do that, it's enough to perform a kinesiology test, besides there are machines that cost ten times less for that purpose."

I, in short, discover that I bought BICOM only to diagnose, completely forgetting the curative and therapeutic aspect, and I am now aware that diagnosis is only the tip of the iceberg in terms of what this alternative medicine instrument can do.

This innovate electromagnetic research methodology opens future, trusty horizons; it is considered as alternative medicine in Italy, while also being unknown, whereas in Germany it is an integral part of the universal national health care service.

Food, medicines, plants, flours, stones, metals, BICOM can check the magnetic emanation from everything.

In addition, all human organisms have their own frequency, that can be measured and re-set with the help of the bio-resonance.

Magnetic bio-resonance tests with the relative reset of frequencies can be carried out on each composed or simple cellular organism, because they aren't invasive on any level.

When Bicom goes into resonance with an electromagnetic frequency that is tied to an allergy, you can eliminate the problem by using the same frequency with the opposite sign: this doesn't just happen at times, or if you're lucky. It always happens.

Most people have an allergen in their organic cycle.

Every good self-respecting study course has a coffee Break, and it is during this break that I test myself.

Not having undergone any treatment yet, I show some of my classmates, mainly doctors, that I am allergic to beef and that I have a massive milk intolerance.

When the class resumes, I ask what I can do to help my son who has had an anaphylactic shock caused by eating kiwi.

Following my question, the German professor just kept shaking his head. From the simultaneous translation I understand that whet he it was kiwi or something else, that didn't matter, or rather, kiwi was only the outbreak element: the fuse.

Today it may be kiwi; tomorrow it will be a different food.

What we need to find is the dynamite.

What the teacher wants me to understand is the reaction to a heavy metal, that Federico's body keeps in intercellular spaces under the guise of scoria, toxin, intolerance, incompatibility or other.

He explains to me that together with the recording instruments for the machine, there are also the necessary instruments to discover, deactivate and dispose of it.

Using the vials I own, I only need to identify the negative elements, treat them all together, invert the frequencies, repeat the treatment once a week for even four or five times, until everything is fixed.

With the original BICOM vials, the matter could be solved in one or at most two sittings.

The treatment, besides, has a prolonged effect, it may happen that over the years something goes off parameter again, but in a lighter form. In that case it is sufficient to repeat the treatment in the same way.

The cure consists in connecting the negative elements going in, to the opening of a container or to the vial container, and then connecting the patient with two outgoing wires that have two small brass balls at the end, balls that the patient must hold in his hands.

This is how messages are sent to the body in exam. They are received by the hand cells and transmitted to the cells of the entire organism. This noninvasive treatment takes a few minutes, it doesn't provoke any sensitization, and it causes no collateral effect.

The topic for the following day was the BICOM set of five elements.

I had bought this set to test on Federico and myself and I didn't make much use of it with other people.

The set of the five elements is based on Chinese Medicine: on complete domain, the peripheral movement and on the balanced redistribution of energy.

Each element has a pseudonym denomination and is paired with some of the main colors we find in nature:

Fire is red, associated with about ten meridians, including the heart, the small intestine and circulation.

Water is blue associated with kidneys, the bladder and allergies.

Metal is white and associated with lungs, the bronchial tubes, skin and the connective tissue.

Earth is yellow and associated with the stomach, spleen, pancreas and the nervous system.

Wood is green and associated with liver and articulations.

Each column of groups and subgroups that builds the set of five elements is formed by multiple vials, that represent the different organs.

When there's a problem, an organ consumes more energy. This can be observed with the bio magnetic resonance test.

The detected drop in potential total energy causes a loss of energy in another organ of the same color.

Sometimes the organ loses a moderate amount of energy, other times a significant amount.

When things become serious, one element subtracts energy from another element, thereby upsetting the balance of the entire organism and making it fertile ground for many diseases, sometimes serious.

At first, Federico's profile showed inconsistency with the water element, the light blue color that has allergies and kidneys as meridian, but not skin, that is instead associated with the meridian of the lungs.

The more I follow the course of alternative medicine, and specifically the magnetic bio resonance, the more feel like I'm going in the right direction.

During the previous years, in spite of all the amount of vital strength, trips, specialist examinations, treatments, medicines and more, Federico experienced no visible improvement.

This unusual, irritating and, for the moment, scarcely curable illness, had never allowed him any respite, almost taking away from him the chance of living a normal life like kids his own age; continuously obliging him to small sacrifices and to live outside the traditional mould of a human being.

I realize I must do everything possible to bring my son's life back to normal.

Sitting in a room, with the light of just one candle, that's placed on the wall shelf where my father often kept his wax matches with a few loose cigarettes, I realize how much and for how many times human thought has travelled with approximation.

We never really managed to erase our ancestral concerns, but above all, we have hardly ever found a solution to the many enigmas that reduce the fairness of a quiet life.

The light suddenly weakens, a sudden draught flattens the flame, lighting up the wall of the room.

Such is the feeling with our hopes: we know little, and we are often in a scarcely lit room.

I often looked for the solution to the problem that afflicted Federico, but I was in the dark. Sometimes hope needs to be cultivated too: the candle flame moves again and this time the room takes on different tones. It's enough to follow the gush of wind, maybe hope will be lit again.

Dawn is coming, night is ending, and this war is not won, but every battle needs to be always supported by innovation. This is what makes us superior: the ability to evolve and find the right way in the calm sea moments.

I did a lot of searching during all this time, and perhaps the machine that uses frequencies can replace the candle.

I put out the candle, I am tired, I'll go and rest a little.

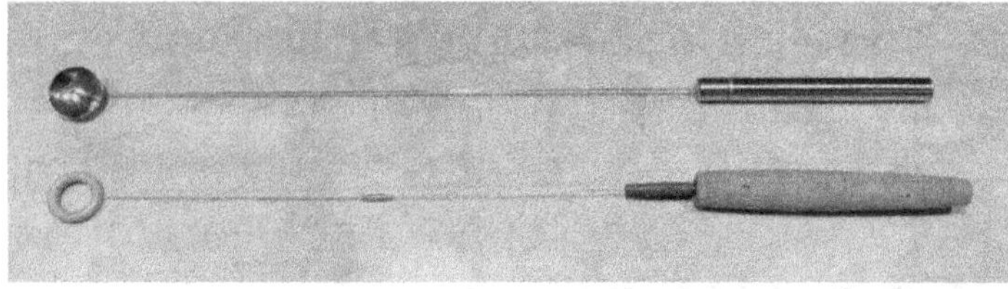

BIREK

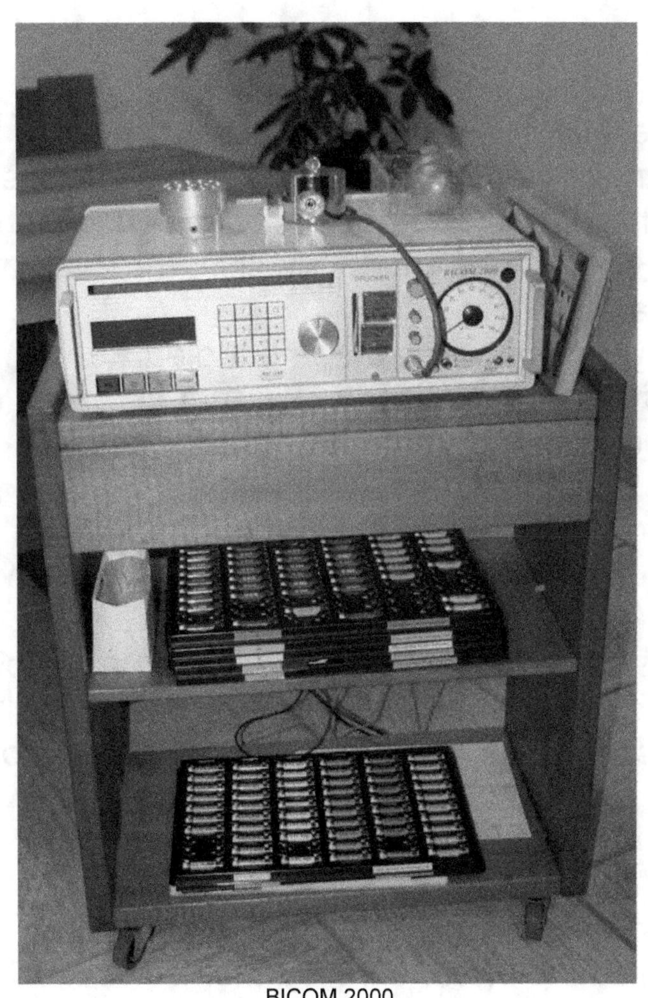

BICOM 2000

Chapter VII

My brother is eight years younger than me and I remember that when he was little he had skin problems, mainly on his cheeks. Up until age three his hands were partially restrained, so that he could not scratch himself and further irritate his skin, that was already weak and in precarious state.

He was nine years old when our father died.

My mother and I took care of him so that he got at least the needed education. In the following years he got a diploma as an electronic expert.

Since his adolescence, together with some school friends, he was involved in volunteering and philanthropy, and he was a dedicated member of the organization "Mato Grosso".

This movement -- through free labor aimed at helping the poor and unprivileged – offered young people the chance to have a formative experience outside of the methodic and capitalistic context of Western countries.

In Italy the boys collected paper, glass and metal scrap to finance the missions.

The ones who worked the hardest, or who felt they had an inner calling to know something more, enrolled themselves for a 4 month period of work in a mission in South America.

In the meantime I found him a job with a mechanical company, the owner being a friend of mine.

In the summer of 1982 he went for 4 months to Chacas in Peru where there was a woodworker and carving school for boys who were chosen because they were among the most marginalized and poor of the area.

It was the year of the football world championship.

I remember Italy's winning match which was followed with great enthusiasm both in homeland and abroad.

Among the girls who were members of the Mato Grosso operation he met and married Nicoletta.

In 1987he changed his job and went to the Rivadossi workshop. There he was a furniture artist who sent his furniture and carving designs to Peru for further production.

The following year together with his wife and son Francesco, who was only two years old at the time, he went to live in Peru.

In the caving school they produced furniture using excellent wood and created handwork and carvings without using nails.

From then onwards he made continuous flights to Peru. In Latin America his two other children were Giovanni and Simone, were born.

On a rare visit back to Italy, I went to pick them up from the airport in Milan and then drove them to their grandparents.

The first thing that their grandmother did was to take little Simone wash him well. I can still see that little baby running away naked from his grandmother's arms towards his mother Nicoletta and shouting with irrational wonder: "Mamma, mamma come and see! Hot water is flowing down from the tap!"

Bruno, my brother, while working in the woodworking department, had aggravated his allergy problems.

While he was in Peru he felt well but on returning to Italy, he often had red eyes and was exhausted from continuously sneezing.

With the special food diet which I suggested to him he felt physically better, but when I treated him with the bio resonance allergy treatment, he felt reborn.

The families of the "Mato Grosso" boys are very united and generally had many children; it was easy for my brother to convince his friends to expose all their families to my allergy tests.

Things advanced to the point where I began to treat people, and this circle expanded to include parents, brothers, friends and their children.

This group of people, almost a large crowd, allowed me to analyze them giving me full medical access. This further allowed me to make a serious data collection, which later bore fruit.

I bought a lot of furniture for my house, all of which come from Peru, so that when anyone came for a test or treatment, looking around my house they felt at home, and it was easier for me, to continue questioning without anybody being afraid of being misunderstood.

I managed to help and many resolved cases were particularly valued in the volunteer workers' families; as for example the one of the young mother whose 10 year old child had allergic asthma, with an often worrying respiratory crisis.

The test results showed the typical pollen, plant and an unusual goose feather allergy.

I started the test treatment. One month later, the child's mother told me that her son definitely felt better.

He no longer suffered from continuous nights of urination and bed-wetting; things she had not told me before the treatment. She asked me kindly if I could see her nephew.

A pensioner who worked voluntarily with the "Mato Grosso" foundation, came to me with allergy problems.

I initiated the treatment without thinking about any other risk although a big red birthmark was prominent between his nose and one eye.

He had booked a place in the local hospital for the removal of that same skin blemish. However, the day after the allergy treatment his birthmark had begun to peel off and several days later, it had completely disappeared. So he cancelled the operation.

The O.M.G (Mato Grosso) association has different volunteers who continue the mission in South America for a period of two or three years.

When they return to a change of diet they are also exposed to dust and pollen which initiate many allergy problems. I have checked many similar people who had to stay for a period in hospital, noticing various intolerances amongst others to pork meat. This was a common grievance almost all patients.

After a strict food diet and two sessions of treatments these patients felt much better.

My work has had an enormous resonance. I began to receive people of every nationality belonging to the most diverse voluntary associations, all wanting the same thing; to be tested, to receive the appropriate therapy and at long last to be cured from irritating and oppressive allergies which had never definitively been eradicated using the traditional medicinal therapy .

I treat everybody gratuitously .

A 22 year old man was a very unusual patient. He had been rushed twice within fifteen days to hospital; once because he had eaten a walnut and the second time because had eaten pasta with pesto.

He was a strong boy with two strong hands. When I discovered a beef allergy it became normal for me to effect the Chinese test.

I did not think it possible that my own delicate employer hands could win over the rough hands of a butcher.

I began the treatment with the different modulations.

After some weeks he confirmed that he felt better.

Moreover, he informed me that he had effected the same Chinese ring test to all his brothers and discovered that his youngest brother had his same food intolerance.

A neighbour with his father came to see us at our house in the mountains.

"It is a difficult period for us," the girl confessed to me.

"My mother died in spite of all cures, chemotherapy included. My father is a pensioner with Parkinson's disease. He is always very tired and if it were not for me, he would never get up from his bed. This is making me very worried.

Her father was the first person with Parkinson's disease who had given me the possibility of testing this illness; it made me particularly interested.

During the five element test the result showed a high level of heavy metals; the other ampoules signaled cobalt and palladium presence.

Alarmed I immediately used the same test on his daughter who didn't show any problem.

Then I exposed her father to several other treatments to eliminate the heavy metal presence and in addition I also tried a treatment for his depression.

When I came back from vacation in the mountains I brought with me a basket of mushrooms which had been picked by the girl's father. By walking through the countryside to look for mushrooms it seemed as if he had again found his old vigor and passion for life.

The fact that the father's body was full of palladium while his daughter's was not, pulled me up short. Two doubts obsessed me: The first was; I was working in close contact with people who having had a chemotherapy treatment could absorb in one way or other the harmful magnetism or passive degeneration caused by the heavy metals used in this treatment.

The second was that because the male sex was frailer, he had kept these heavy metals for long.

So I spoke about it to a friend of mine who had had a bone marrow transplant after doctors had used the same related cures.

He had lost his grey hair that was now growing back again. I checked him and noticed the same heavy metal content. So I called his brother, who worked with him, and found a predominant absorption of palladium and cobalt when I subjected him the treatment.

The brother brought the rest of his family to me for testing but the result was negative.

In the same office another male employee also worked.

As soon as possible I also tested him and again with the same results. He also showed up positive by having in his organism a big dose of heavy metals. I also treated him.

Finally, I checked the family of a friend of mine. The three boys had palladium and cobalt traces, but his wife and the daughter did not.

Following this lead, I checked a relative of my wife who had undergone a breast operation following chemotherapy.

Immediately, the first test came out a clear palladium and cobalt presence.

I started the treatment, but unfortunately her arms, the relative articulations, wrists, elbows and shoulders hurt her very much. It was very difficult for her to hold the two spheres in her hands.

As we continued with the treatment, the pain became less. I visited her at home with the ampoules, I also checked her husband who had tested to heavy metals while his daughters had not. The husband didn't want to do any treatment.

I also happened to verify an old couple. The husband showed signs of palladium while his wife did not. His wife had been operated on ten years earlier because of a breast tumor. She had also undergone chemotherapy but showed no residues of heavy metal.

I also found palladium and cobalt traces in two priests who had visited the sick undergoing chemotherapy treatment. One day at the exit of the hospital, my wife met a young boy who lived in our town. He had not felt very well at work and while he was at the bank he blacked out. He was hospitalized for some days, but the reason for his collapse was never found.

My wife knew that the boy's mother had undergone long intensive chemotherapy treatment for the presence of bony timorous cells. I invited him to be treated for the relative tests with my bio resonance equipment.

During the test palladium and cobalt traces showed up. Again for this case I made the relevant treatment and invited the boy to also bring his father to the sessions.

I also noticed the same thing in a sprightly pensioner who didn't show any particular symptoms.

But I wasn't calm. Of the family members under examination only the son-in-law who lived on the upper floor of the same house was missing.

After some months I met the young banker, who in the meantime did not show any more leipothymic symptoms. I completed my scientific curiosity about the medical connection between family members towards the tests. I suggested that he introduce me as soon as possible to also test his sister, her husband and their two daughters.

As I suspected, traces of palladium and cobalt were found only in the male members to whom I made the treatment. The case of Parkinson's disease showed a nickel allergy. The first time I saw this man I had to keep repeating my questions two or three times in order to get an answer. After the treatment he still complained about various health problems but I found him definitely more awake. Other Parkinson's disease case involving an older person also showed a nickel allergy, who however, was very lucid even if he claimed to become tired very quickly. I tested him with his hand.

Before undergoing treatment he was easily tired and without energy. After the treatment and cure, even if he exhibited a delicate constitution, he could still manage to hold the rings with greater force.

Some days later he brought me his niece who had a pollen allergy. I also noticed a nickel allergy even in two cases of multiple sclerosis which I tested. When I practiced the treatment to eliminate the heavy metals, both felt better but this wellbeing remained only for some days. The Alzheimer case faired better.

Also in this patient there was presence of nickel allergy.

After the treatment I heard from her two children that the octogenarian lady was calmer, and during the night had slept better than previously when she had suffered from insomnia.

A person who began to climb up along the mountain path waved to me. By now it was getting dark so I decided to go quickly. Shall I retrace my steps or shall I follow the mysterious man who even if far away looked as if he knew me very well? He seemed to know my body language to communicate with the likes of me.

I was feeling strangely calm and hungry.

Looking at the sky I could see some mountain falcons.

I could feel good sensations through my body. The Navajos would say "buon presagio" (a good omen).

The falcons were turning around taking advantage of the thermal upward draught without beating a wing. In the sky they formed a big eight, yes… buon presagio,….

Surely buon presagio.

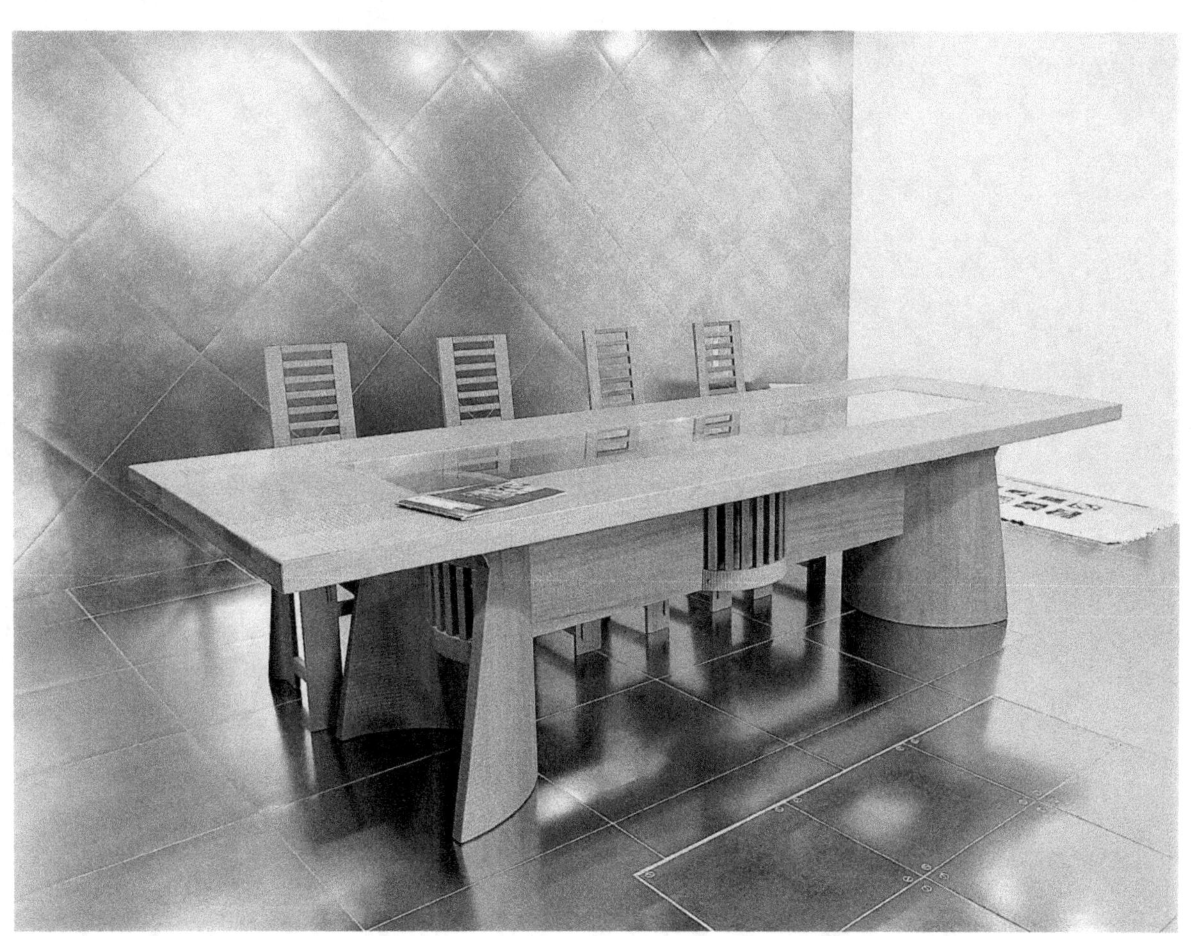

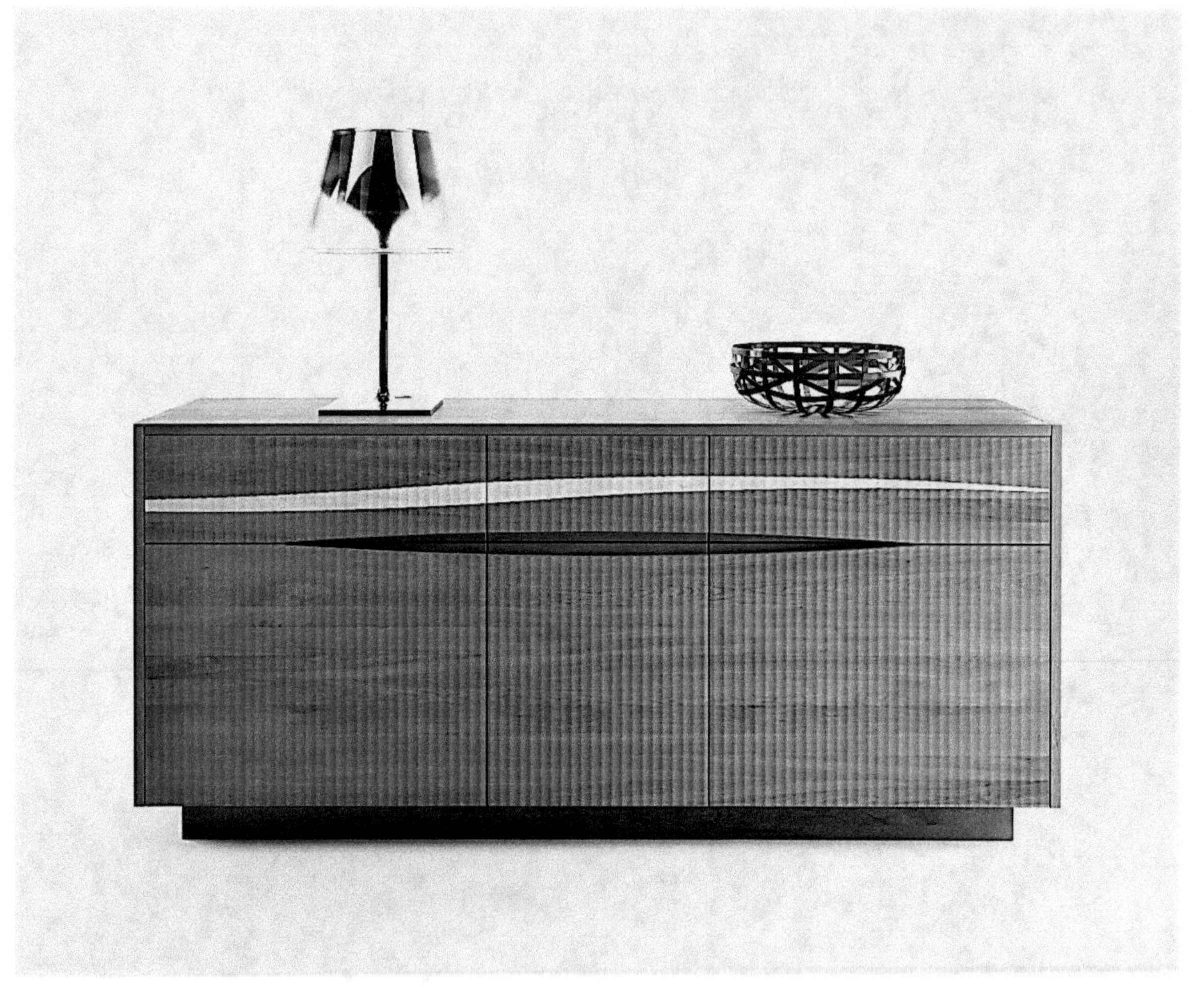

Peruvian Furniture

Chapter VIII

I have always known I was a decidedly strange and original type, but I reached the pinnacle of my eccentricity when, after having attended the chromo therapy course, I could not find the right shirts as I had become excessively overweight, so I went to a shirt maker and asked him to make me 10 bespoke shirts all yellow, even if they came in two different tonalities.

My constant stomachache found a bit of comfort with the yellow color.

One day a lady who had asthma problems often leading to a breathing crisis, came to me. I tested her for many things, including foods, without discovering anything. I then continued with powders and pollens but yet again - nothing.

The woman confessed to me that an increased downward trend had begun several days prior, together with the presence of the colored primroses added as ornament to the living-room windows.

At this point the mental connection was very easy with the ampoules, which seldom gave a patient a negative result.

These are consequently not used very much as a primary allergy test as there are others with regard to flowers of different typologies.

This time, the unusual set showed a strong primrose allergy.

In the same week my nephew Simone complained about the presence of red spots.

I had previously treated him for a strong psoriasis on his hands, I asked the child's mother and got immediate confirmation: there were yellow primroses in the house, in a big Peruvian bowl.

Both patients underwent treatment with the electromagnetic bio resonance with inverted waves and this problem was also happily resolved with a positive outcome.

Later, a bank executive told me that his infant child had spots over his whole body. I checked his baby and found a strong food intolerance for cow milk.

I suggested they substitute cow's milk for goat milk and in a couple of days all the spots had completely disappeared.

A few months after, he told me that he had gone skiing for a week, and as he couldn't find any goat milk he gave him cow milk, and the child was immediately full of spots.

Another ex-colleague told me that his wife often had a rash of red spots covering her whole body and that caused her constant itching.

He also told me that, as she was a celiac, all the products she ate had to be bought at the drugstore.

Following our conversation these products were brought to me. They were made in Germany and in Italy.

I carried out the test on all the German products which were good and tested positive, while two out of four Italian products tested negative.

The skin rash disappeared within three days, so I suggested to the lady that she refer this matter to her family doctor, while also offering him a chance of seeing the machine with which we had done the tests. From my side I was completely at his disposal.

The lady was very disappointed when her family doctor told her that he was not interested in the machine and that he did not want any interference with his regular practice.

At that point, I tried to test on myself the incriminating products which the lady had left on the table.

As I found them negative, I then tested them on my wife and other relatives and obtained the same result.

I did not know what these products contained, but how can any food be noxious for one person while everybody else can use it with impunity?

I tested some foreigners and I discovered that those who came from Eastern European countries like Romanians, Moldavians, Ukrainians, much like Chinese and Pakistanis, were 90% egg intolerant; Africans and inhabitants of the Caribbean are for the main part cow milk intolerant.

I've treated an Argentinean together with his Italian wife.

He had moved to Spain after the Argentinean financial crisis. He was beef intolerant and allergic to olives.

Previously I had treated his son who had told me about his father .

He proposed I go to Spain in order to treat many other people.

He suggested that I could make a fortune with all the beef and olive allergies that are widespread in Spain.

Among those who had helped me in my research, there was a chemist who sold high quality homeopathic products.

The chemist produced tablets and creams by order. Among the best products he had were some pro biotic enzymes whose great effectiveness I had verified.

They are milk enzymes and thus not suitable for those who are milk intolerant. For such people there are milk-free products or over the counter products like "Enterogermina".

During one particular part of my research using homeopathic products, the chemist gave me all the available products he had, for free.

Dedicating two afternoons to my research, I poured over hundreds of products in ampoules and then carried the test out on about thirty people.

It was with big disappointment that I noticed that only two or three of all these tested products were definitely positive in effect, while more than twenty were negative: the rest were neutral, namely they were neither good nor bad.

In my wife's case they were all negative because they were conserved in a mother tincture with an alcoholic base. She is alcohol intolerant; she never drank a glass of bubbly, not even at birthdays or on New Year's Eve.

The machine (BICOM) does not accept complex products and so I couldn't use these ampoules for the treatments, be it the negative or the positive ones.

Regarding the low percentage of tested products that proved positive, I spoke with my chemist friend who told me: "I would marvel if it proved the opposite.

These products are all effective medicines so they must be taken when necessary, prescribed by a doctor or chemist, and not suggested by relatives and friends."

In particular, there was a product that I found to be negative for most people; a pain-killer called "Devil Claw".

I continued testing these products.

Among those I often found positive, I can affirm that the magnesium was always good, and Echinacea was always indicated for asthma and pollens.

A retired lady came to me bringing with her a jar of aloe.

She had gotten it from her daughter who had benefited from using it. I took a test with the Birek and verified that the product tested noxious for her while it proved innocuous on me.

I tasted the product and noticed the presence of honey, and I had seen from the phials that the woman was honey intolerant.

Whenever there is a negative component, the whole composition becomes negative.

My son was milk intolerant, so I had to eliminate pasta that contained milk and eliminate ham because some of it was boiled in milk.

An intolerance for certain kinds of fruit is very common.

It can happen that a person can be kiwi intolerant but not banana intolerant. Or again, a person can react to eating peaches but not to apples and vice versa.

And eating a fruit salad is the worst possible thing that a person with a fruit intolerance can do.

A friend of mine who was skeptical of my findings told me that he would believe in the potential of my machine only if I could cure an acquaintance of his.

As agreed, one afternoon he presented a 27 year old man to me whose face was completely spoiled from psoriasis.

"I'm so careful with my hygiene. I take a shower twice a day in the morning and again in the evening.

My mother changes the bed sheets each day and every two weeks I get a cortisone injection which is effective for short time.

I got the last one injection two days ago", he said to me, depressed.

"I have tried everything, even the cream used in Switzerland for sensitive cow tits", he continued sadly

showing that he believed his to be a hopeless case.

I began to cure the allergies to nickel, pollens, grasses and dust mites.

I saw he had a milk and Solanaceae intolerance, so I recommended that he regularly drank mineral water and avoid milk, potatoes, tomatoes and all other natural products that contained these substances, and to come back in two weeks.

A fortnight later he told me that he felt much better.

As of that day, he had not needed any cortisone injection and his mother had not had to change his bed sheets so frequently.

This second time I cured him for his stomachache, too.

His metabolism showed a marked energetic lack of balance.

When he came back he was delighted. He did not need the cortisone injection anymore. However, because he was very stressed out, I decided to cure his stress and tension with the BICOM phial, getting them back to a balanced equilibrium using the right energetic magnetism.

After the treatment, he informed me of a car accident he had had, and that before his psychosomatic readjustment with the BICOM machine he might have reacted very badly, in all probability by fighting with the driver.

Now he was surprised how much he could control himself; even smiling while compiling a simple form for an assessment of the damage.

This was his spontaneous story.

During the next few days I constantly monitored him.

The skin on his face began to lighten even if the signs of the psoriasis were still very deep.

At this point with the use of special impulses I gave the right information to the connective tissue cells for a rapid healing of the scar tissues.

I suggested that he took a holiday at the sea side.

When he came back from his beach holiday his face as well as his body were completely healed.

He thanked me with an emotional voice.

I explained to him that I did this only and exclusively for research and completely free of charge.

He did not want to hear any explanation and with much euphoria repeated to me many times the words thank you. And then, I understood the reason for his deep gratitude, as he explained to me that finally, like all guys his age, he could now manage to find a girlfriend.

As he repeated this last sentence, I felt a strong sensation, that welled from my stomach up to my eyes.

A strange and powerful warm sense of wellbeing took hold of me. The monster -- that was his nickname -- moved me, he really moved me.

A family friend who had a passion for bikes, complained that he had backache and he had had it for several months.

After having invited him many times to come to my house, I finally found him at a ceremony. When we had finished eating he asked me: "Is the invitation for the cure still valid?"

"I'm going home now; if you want to come with me I can make a treatment for you immediately", I replied.

I told him to take off his ring and place it together with the clock and his mobile phone on the table.

Then I started with the tests.

As the machine made the usual tone to signify that the therapy was ending, his mobile phone rang. Quickly he gave me back the balls for the magnetic transduction, sprang up and answered the call.

Then he asked me: "Why are you laughing?" "I'm laughing because earlier you told me that you had difficultly standing up, and just now you sprang up without any problem," I answered him.

He stood up and sat down several times. "I don't feel a thing any-more."

"Now don't exaggerate, otherwise you will get backache again." I said jokingly to him.

The mother of my son's school friend suffered from headaches.

When she heard by chance from an acquaintance that she could be cured by the machine for her headaches, my son's school friend asked me if he could bring his mother to be cured.

The lady had suffered from different pollen allergies which the set of five elements showed by tests on her stomach.

The first therapy was the basic one, followed by the other two.

I was not able to obtain the desired outcome. The headache symptoms worsened, but the results of the allergic tests prescribed by the doctor at this point gave completely negative results.

One day somebody asked me to check their child who was two years old and had always suffered from dysentery.

They had been on holiday in Tunis, and during the holiday the child had essentially only drunk milk.

The test results showed an intolerance for wheat.

At that point I checked the parents and I discovered that the father had the same intolerance.

He, however, had often complained about headaches.

After two treatment sessions the intolerance had receded but he still showed all the other intestinal problems.

An overweight girl who wanted to lose weight had followed a rigid diet with some of the meals consisting only of fruit and vegetables.

I checked her, and discovered that she had an intolerance to all fruit.

By eliminating the fruit, but eating all other food normally she quickly lost her excess weight.

A boy who weighed over 120 kg, continued to put on weight. From the analysis I saw that he was solanaceae plant intolerant which could be potatoes, tomatoes and many other vegetables.

When he eliminated those, he felt decidedly better.

Now the hawks moved their flying pattern, they were near the top of the mountain.

It was difficult for me to see them, they were far away.

While I could well distinguish the figure with the raised Collar, he showed me by pointing with the finger of his right hand to the sky where the farthest hawks were flying.

This looked like an invitation for me to rise higher.

I felt that this was the right moment to move, I made a waiting gesture and started walking towards the beginning of the inaccessible pathway.

I really did not know what I was going to do by following the figure. I did not know back then, but I was sure that the person wanted to go higher and had found a good friend.

The love for challenge is my best gene. I was sure that because of my prosthesis it would be much more difficult to reach him, but I knew that the road had begun and that I wanted to continue through, until I had reached the top, with or without a friend.

In the meantime, a luminous moon began to shine from behind the mountain top, the limpid light spreading and making long shadows that seemed threatening and unsettling.

I had seen worse things in my life and I had experienced many more worries than these.

I continued to walk, trying to accelerate my stride, an irritating pain coming from my hip, …. Straight ahead, …you always have to keep going straight ahead.

Chapter IX

I have always had a congenital illness in my hips; my sister on the other hand has never experienced any problem till she was 45 years old, when her physique suffered a massive vertical collapse.

Within one year she was not able to walk anymore and had strong aches and pains on her right hip, even when she made the slightest movement.

When she had the first operation on the femur the graft prosthesis caused her an irreversible fracture of the pelvis.

Starting from then on, eleven surgeries followed, one after the other, ten on the right leg and one on the left leg.

When I bought BICOM, I thought both of her and Federico, whom in the meantime I had completely cured of every form of psoriasis, finally freeing himself of all the other allergies that had bothered his life as a young boy.

I ardently desired to relieve a bit of my sister's unexpected suffering.

I also thought that I had to have some practical but effective means of transport for my machine when it was necessary, including the enclosed convent where my sister had decided to remain for the rest of her life.

For this reason I asked my brother together with his volunteers to build a trolley out of a special type of South American wood, the kaoba.

The structure was built and kept together without using any nails, in order to avoid whatever interference might occur between the metals, and in order to avoid allergic interactions with European plants.

With this trolley I went to Milan to cure my sister.

Furthermore, before I began the treatment, I had told her to go on a diet. Then I cured her of all the hereditary allergies which were the same as mine.

Following her first treatment session, after having bought a new phial set suitable for more tests, I could finally cancel the side effects of the numerous rounds of anesthesia she had undergone in such a short time.

My sister told me that when she sat at the computer, after about ten minutes she felt her leg going numb and had to stop working.

When I also came in possession of a new set of phials for an environmental magnetic recording, I noticed a consistent allergy to plastic. I cured her with excellent results that surpassed all my expectations regarding this problem.

Within her community, there were also some nuns who were allergic to pollen.

Each time I visited her I brought the machine with me while she brought lots of patients to see me.

These sisters have received many benefits and complete healing against the classical allergy pathologies.

Spring with its many different blossoms and flowers was not a problem anymore, even if in autumn a couple of nuns had relapses.

Among those who experienced a relapse, there was a sister who had previously undergone many traditional allergy tests, that underlined she was ambrosia allergic.

This is a type of grass that blossoms only during the summer.

This plant does not grow near us, so I could not treat the patient if I could not get a sample or a phial for the magnetic recording.

Some days afterwards, I received a telephone call from my sister who told me that the ambrosia plant had been found and could the patient come to me at home in order to start the treatment.

No problem I replied, checking the plant, the flower and the leaves.

I noticed that the leaves gave a stronger resonance when tested, so I inserted the leaves in a phial and I started the treatment with effective results.

My sister underwent surgery at Ravenna, Marseille and Florence, but it was a renowned professor from the Gaetano Pini Clinic in Milan who got her walking again.

But unfortunately all these operations had short-lived benefits, and for that reason after the last operation I activated an energetic preparation treatment on my sister Carla.

During the last operation on my sister I had not found on her any problems caused by the anesthetic and after a short rehabilitation period she was sent to a convent where there were sisters who were older and sicker than she was.

She had hardly arrived at this convent when I received a telephone call from her. She wanted me to visit her immediately because she needed me and my machine.

"Heh, not so fast, I only saw you last week and the machine didn't show anything peculiar; and then we also have to check the medicines you must take, and test whether they're positive for you."

I told her.

"But it is not for me!"

"I found an old school friend and she is a nurse here in this institute. She is full of spots all over her arms. I've never seen anything like it. I think it must be a strong allergy reaction of some sort," she replied.

So the following Saturday I went to Contra, a really relaxing place, situated on the hills and surrounded by meditative centuries-old plants.

I completed the tests that told me there was a massive presence of hard metals, especially palladium and cobalt.

I asked the nurse if she had ever undergone chemotherapy treatment.

"No I haven't, but it's my job to transport by car, the nuns who need this kind of treatment and honestly this disturbs me a bit."

She answered.

I completed the treatment and the spots went away within a short amount of time.

My sister advised me to come back and visit her with the machine as soon as possible because in the same hospice there was a lay nurse who also had similar spots and most probably the test would give the same results.

By now I had won everybody's confidence, in particular, the confidence of one of the nurses. She asked me to check an old patient who had many problems including insomnia and who complained so much during the night, that she bothered the other patients in the institute.

She had allergic problems due to pollens, so I checked the medicines she was taking, and among them were products which had given particularly negative results.

It was a common procedure and the nurse let me check a similar product which to my surprise had tested positive.

What was the difference between the two products?

The first was a product that could be gotten for free under the National Health Service, while the second had to be paid for and prescribed by an appropriate doctor.

At this point it was only necessary to eliminate the medicine and complete the treatment with the negative magnetic resonance. The effect was amazing. After only two days the patient was able to sleep throughout

the night, and during day hours, she was far more active and receptive.

In another case a patient had problems because of a tumor and had to be operated on again.

My set of tests gave me no negative signal showing no damaged cells.

I told the nurse, and she also confirmed that the traditional examinations had not shown any illness, the operation being part of a prevention program.

A relative of my wife's was diagnosed with a problem and on the basis of this diagnosis was told she had to undergo surgery.

The lady was not as convinced as the doctors, and asked me for an opinion. I told the lady specifically that this was not my job but if she wanted, I could carry out a test with the Birek machine. The test confirmed the presence of damaged cells and so I suggested to the worried patient to trust the doctors.

There was also a 40 year old man who told me that his whole body hurt him. I made the five elements test and found the main bio magnetic imbalance was in the zone of mastication; to be more precise it was localized in his teeth. I asked him when was the last time he had visited the dentist. "Never," was his reply.

At this point it was not necessary to make any helpful treatment.

I met him some weeks later and when he came near to me he said, "You brought me bad luck. Two days after I met you I made an appointment with the dentist.

He checked two teeth but treated me for four!"

"You don't think that within two days a further two teeth can decay, do you?" I replied.

I met a young couple whose small child had always experienced respiratory problems.

The problems had started in September. The little girl had only gone to Kindergarten for a few days when she became ill and was forced to stay home during the month of October as well. It was in November that medical exams took place, along with various tests, which resulted in her being rushed to the local hospital.

From December to February, the little girl did not move out of her home environment and soon began to feel better.

One sunny day the child went into the garden to play, Her parents were horrified to see that all the symptoms came back, and caused several strong asthma attacks.

She was rushed to hospital again but unfortunately there were not many treatments that were able to heal her, and equally few future possible cures.

As the parents already knew that I had cured some children from asthma, they asked me to consider treating their daughter.

The general tests produced a very strong incompatibility for environmental conditions, in particular the child was very allergic to ozone.

It was the first time I had found this element as an allergy. I told to the parents that I had had absolutely no idea about the meaning of this kind of allergy and where it came from.

Anyway I made the ozone detoxification treatment and I promised to inform them about everything I could research about this strange allergy.

Some days afterwards the child's father told me that he also had done some research from which he found out that tuff stones emanate ozone gas.

He also said that in September he had built a new house garden and had used this kind of stone to built a low wall about 60 cm high to follow the path what led inside the house.

At that point he asked me if he had to remove all those stones and remake the garden anew in order to avoid his child's exposure to this allergen.

As I had treated the ozone allergy and had balanced the protection parameters for the element in question, I thought the child should experience no problems.

The treatment was about four minutes long, and could be done again in case it was necessary.

Since then two years have gone by, and I have not seen them again.

A lady who lived near my father's house, told me that she had a hyperactive son who caused major embarrassment.

When I saw him for the first time I only made some food tests and found nothing especially alarming but when I bought the new sets I asked to see him again so that I could carry out some new tests on him.

The mother gave me permission to test him but only for two minutes, during which I registered a moderate nickel allergy.

As I could not oblige her to treat her son with my therapeutic method, I left.

Following this initial meeting I was informed that her son's problem had increased alarmingly.

From a personal research I discovered another small child, this time from Milan, who had been given the same diagnosis of hyperactivity.

He had been treated with strong sedatives which were regularly given to him.

So I spoke with the small patient's aunt who told me more about this matter. I gave her the address of the pediatrician in Milan who used the bio-resonance as a regular therapy. I knew through her that this Hippocrates supporter successful cured the child.

Chapter X

During a further refresher course I met the German professor again, who asked me how things were going. He was surprised that I could carry out tests and treatments for the most part only on allergy subjects.

He explained that this machine was also able to control the yin and yang energetic status and to verify the biological conditions of the different body organs.

Many programs could control treatment without using the phials, the frequency being enough to cure cicatrix, adhesion, depression, freeing the backbone from energetic blocks and to better the absorption of proteins and acids.

As the course got underway, among the many different arguments formulated, questions arose about celiac disease. We were all surprised and the German professor was amazed when he discovered that in Italy celiac disease is not curable and that the health service only gives special food as a treatment.

During the course we were given a lecture that had to be a stimulus for the participating colleagues to undertake research and find confirmation of the practical use and medical potentiality of the electromagnetic bio resonance.

In the following days I again read the handbooks, especially those concerning treatment that do not require the use of phials. Then I started to test scars, verify the status of depression, ictus and much more.

In order to get a closer look at research examination and in order to increase my own personal knowledge, I decided to participate to a conference about the coeliac disease which was taking place at the University of Medicine in Brescia.

There, the speaker expressed amazement referring to the acquisition of data which annually gave the number of coeliac disease registered in the territory of our province of Brescia, approximately one per thousand, against four per thousand at the national average.

For me, all these results were undeniably consistent with information extracted from the tests done during these years of research thanks to the co-operation of the electromagnetic bio resonance.

From my personal experience in this specific research Field, particularly regarding food intolerances, I can confirm that all the inhabitants coming from the valley of Brescia who were blood relations, as well as for the most part other people I examined, had shown a good wheat tolerance and were thus less subject to coeliac disease.

I had tested a family who between them showed evidence of intolerance problems for the well known graminaceae plant, the father who had celiac disease also exhibited a kind of psoriasis, while his daughter with the same pathology showed no signs on her skin tissue.

A young woman of thirty told me how her coeliac disease started.

Because she had mastication problems, she had undergone important and delicate mouth surgery.

For obvious reasons she was then forced to modify all the ingredients of her normal diet, eating only fluid food which did not include bread or pasta.

When she eventually started eating normally again she also consumed regular portions of bread and pasta but then came her stomach problems, followed by the diagnosis of coeliac disease.

At that point of my research I only carried out allergy tests on my patients, the majority of them showing celiac disease and an intolerance towards wheat and corn associated with approximately another 30 foods of different nature.

Publicity, by now well ascertained, can sell different types of foods with a not always identifiable quality, to a large variety of people.

This in itself is serious enough but it gains greater importance when you can sell products of dubious value or absolute harm to a normal consumer who has inside themselves the celiac disease.

It is also well known that grandfathers are the most easily influenced heads of the family when it comes to a question of good health and complete wellbeing of their grandchildren.

Almost punctually, an old lady came to me in my studio with her grandchild who was approximately five years old.

The Birek confirmed classic wheat Intolerance, but then began vibrating strongly to the horizontal and was forcefully negative when I verified a particular type of rice chocolate that was regularly sold at the chemist's as a so called integrated alimentary product for coeliac people.

So I got up and went into the kitchen and took a normal piece of 75% dark chocolate. This irreproachable and highly thought of sweet antidepressant began occupying space in our refrigerator when Federico was put on a diet for his serious intolerances.

Using the chocolate bar that I had just taken from the refrigerator, the Birek now gave an intensive vertical sign, thus very positive.

I have always thought that chocolate gave a particular predisposition for fun and hilarity but I surely did not expect that once tasted it could bring tears of joy even after nibbling only a little piece.

Among one of the very first cases my sister had brought to me, was a nun who suffered from many different problems, including the presence of big brown spots that covered her whole body and that were decidedly more evident on her arms.

This particular sister taught in Milan and said that besides this problem, she had experienced swellings on her face on multiple occasions.

The worst had happened at Sciacca in Sicily where she went for thermae (thermal water and mud) treatment before going to a convent in Apulia.

Then there was the house on the shore of Lake Como where she went for spiritual exercise and where she felt really ill.

During the test I noticed a heavy nickel and olive allergy; the first only present in the cutlery used during communal meals, while for the second there was no doubt, the places she frequented had a massive presence of olive trees.

I got the confirmation about the results when the nun said with a calm voice, "Now I understand why when I go back home I feel so good. In my family there is the tradition of using silverware when having dinner."

Her intolerance was resolved with excellent results.

I went for a sorrowful visit of condolence because the mother of a girl who participates to the Mato Grosso voluntary work, died during a final operation after having undergone various operations and chemotherapy treatment.

Knowing that her father also had various health problems I invited her to bring him to see me.

A few days later the girl told me her father was not inclined to undergo any kind of treatment.

I felt sorry.

A conversation between this girl and I was followed attentively by another guy who asked me if I could do something for his father who had undergone chemotherapy treatment due to pulmonary problems.

I said that it was better to be in good shape before facing up to that kind of treatment, and told him when I was free, I would visit his father.

During the first appointment I managed to effectively highlight degenerate cells and acarus allergy.

The patient declared that he had respiratory problems and sneezed continuously during the short visit.

I made the treatment with inverted waves for the acarus allergy and an additional supporting cure.

The following month, a few days before the second chemotherapy cycle, the patient came back for the preparation treatment.

At this point I saw that there was no presence of degenerate cells but there were big problems with his metabolism and stomach.

He himself told me that the sneezing fits had reduced in intensity within two or three days and that his respiration was really better as was the reduction both in force and number of his short of breath crisis for missing oxygen, which previously forced him to stop several times while he walked up the stairs.

In the following months the patient felt much better.

Even when the electromagnetic bio resonance machine showed punctual deficiency at the stomach, he did not feel any pain. He even said that his appetite was coming back.

The sister of a relative of mine had been operated for a breast tumor and had great difficulty raising her arms. From my first check it transpired that particular residuals, coming from the anesthesia and a badly healed scar, were sufficient to give her a high level of anxiety and depression.

I completed the cure with inverted waves using the phials of the anesthesia to cure the scar and depression.

During the control visit, the doctors congratulated her on the excellent result of scar healing.

After some time she called me to say, "I've finished the chemotherapy treatment and for four days I've been feeling awful. Can you do something with your machine?"

"If you can come to me I'll try," I replied.

During the treatment to optimize the stomach and metabolism I saw the suffering face of the patient who looked me in the eyes and whispered:

"I feel as if a hand is pushing the high part of my stomach." After treatment her face was visibly happier.

" Now," she said as if by enchantment," I'm feeling the hand releasing its grasp."

This was her direct testimony.

A pensioner from Milan came to me with a red face.

He said, " I renewed my driving license and during the visit they checked my eyesight and hearing. But my problem is with my hands. They are full of arthritis and I can't move them."

His was the first case of smog presence in the organism despite bedrest because of anesthesia, he had various alimentary intolerances, as well as diffuse pollen, graminaceae plant, mites and antioxidant E310 allergies.

I treated all the instabilities with the same power frequency, but this time inverted.

After a few days he called me thanking me, " What makes me very happy is that now I can open and close my hands without any effort."

I have tested, met, known and analyzed a great number of patients since I began my research in the field of alternative medicine.

This multitude of people has been helped by my time, but at the same time the energy of my device and magnetic waves have awarded me many successes in the human field.

I don't want to pontificate about solidarity and it would be superfluous. I just want to restrict all my writing to a sentence of a well known and holy person, " There are ears of corn that are high and nice, but it's often

the curved and less obvious ears of corn that seem to need treatment, but that instead have more grains on them than the other ones.

And it is for that abundant fullness of fruit that they are obliged to curve to complete their full maturity."

Chapter XI

Rising to the top of a mountain, flying over the valleys and plains, feeling the morning breeze brush your face, climbing onto a rough mountain footpath, making a solo crossing to follow the trails of the dolphins in love and more and more and more.

That's exactly how I dreamt when I was a little child.

This handicap on my hips, as if it had been left to me in a will by my family's genetic heredity, caused me to undergo various hip operations in the following years.

During a routine check- up, the surgeon told me there was no hurry to do the surgery, however because of

the family's strong genetic problems he suggested to put me on the back burner and show up when the pain became too strong and hard. It also meant that at night it I would have to be ready to use this new surgical manipulation.

I thought that I had to undergo surgery first on the right leg, but after a couple of years or so, it was the other leg that began to hurt more and more.

I went into hospital for the pre-admission which connected the usual generic visits for confirmation of general good health, blood test and a radiography test at the thorax as well as a cardiogram.

When the heart specialist visited me, I was asked if I had allergies.

On my arm from where the blood sample had been drawn, there was a big bruise showing a swelling of the subcutaneous connective tissue.

The sign of bruising came as no surprise to me and when I got home I immediately used the BICOM's allergy tests to test myself, hoping that the cutaneous irritations were the result of an allergy factor.

The following time I used my car to go to the hospital, I took the bi-rek with me, leaving it in the glove compartment when I returned to the hospital to be re- checked.

From the test results, I noticed an incompatibility with the disinfect-ant used on me during the first analysis .

I put a bit of disinfectant into a phial and went back to the orthopae-dic department to find out more about how the operation would be conducted.

I asked the surgeon if I could check the new prosthesis as I didn't want to become allergic to it.

He answered me politely but letting me know with a calm but marked voice, that he had never heard of cases of allergy in relation to the prosthesis composition elements which would be grafted inside me.

Tantalum and titanium are allergy provoking elements and the pros-thesis would be sealed in a vacuum.

I told the doctor that it would not be necessary for me to open the packing because with the Birek I could check the new prosthesis with-out taking it out of the box.

Holding the disinfectant in one hand, I made the allergy test with the Birek. It gave me negative signs by displaying its characteristically hor-izontal movement lightly vibrating.

At this point the perplexed professor asked me compassionately, "Can I try it too or do you think that my hand will not be sufficiently still?"

The Birek also functioned well in the hands of the well-known surgeon, who nodding his head between disconcertment and disbelief added that we never finish learning.

Before having surgery, I made the pre-operational treatment and then went to the hospital. I paid for a private room and had a peaceful operation.

On the first day I had no fever but on the second day I got fever twice and the third day I had it four times.

That morning I tested myself and with the help of the Birek, I registered a very strong anesthetic residual.

I called my brother and asked him if he could bring me the bio magnetic machine with all the BICOM tools.

I did the treatment of the anesthetic problem and cured the operation scar. Starting from the following day I had no more fever. On the eleventh day they took out the stitches and let me go home three days earlier than scheduled for a natural post operation healing period.

In Brescia I underwent rehabilitation treatment. At home I cured the adhesion and reinforced my tendons, treating my muscles, tendons and ligaments. I continued to repeat this again the following week.

Considering that BICOM continuously gave me the same frequency for each test, during the third week I inserted a chip into myself for it to memorize the reading.

This chip is as big as a two Euro coin and is applied using your fingers by slipping it under your navel and attaching it by means of a special plaster. It continued to repeat the same frequencies without alteration or sequential shift diversion.

That it was emitting something I realized immediately from the second day on, because the skin in contact with the chip became red and gave me a strong sensation of burning.

So I called the agent who suggested to put a piece of gauze between my skin and the chip.

Every day I checked the chip, the Birek was always giving me the vertical positive movement.

This continued for two months more or less.

Meanwhile I tested myself with the five elements but discovered I needed no special treatment.

Everything was solved satisfactorily with less post surgical trauma, good reconstructed scar tissues and above all in an incredibly short space of time; and all this coming from the doctors who were monitoring the check-ups.

It took a long time after this operation before I could go back for the second surgical intervention.

This time they connected me to a small tank which slowly released the pain-killer. This way, I did not

feel the post operational pain as much as I had previously.

The doctors let me go home quickly, being the same team that had previously performed the first operation and telling me that I already knew how to quickly reduce the rehabilitation period.

It is difficult to find a good draught player, but fortunately in the mountains in an apartment close to mine lived my friend Smith.

During the holidays in August we had long interminable challenges; the fact that we were more or less on the same level made playing all the more interesting.

When one of us began to lose more games this invariably meant that he was not feeling well or that he had some problem on his mind.

On one of those days Fausto did not even win one game, so it I asked him almost spontaneously, "What's your problem today? Physical or mental?"

The reply came immediately, "Physical, I have difficulty walking. I have a pain that starts from my back and goes down my right leg to my knee."

"It is better to stop the game and see what the machine can tell us," I replied.

The test of the five elements underlined chemical load and switching from the phials to the set of environmental loadings I found a biphenyl problem.

It was the first time that I had found such an element and during the treatment I asked him what he had done during the day and how he had come in contact with it.

"I was in the yard," he replied " and was welding two things. I used a welding paste but as there was not much work, I did not bother to wear gloves even when it was suggested to always use them when working with this particular paste. A bit of it ended up on my finger but really, it was only a question of one minute.

The following day Fausto brought me the welding paste during the afternoon.

The Birek indication was very negative.

I programmed the machine with inverted waves and within three minutes BICOM gave me the cure which I applied immediately.

After the treatment the Birek did not give me any result.

The day after the treatment Fausto felt really better.

While I was in the mountains again a relative of mine with his wife and daughter came to pay me a visit. I took the opportunity to check the whole family.

My research showed me that they had cavities but that would not stop them from enjoying their holiday.

On the husband I also found a frequency of liver and backbone imbalance.

He confirmed that he constantly had problems with his back.

The wife's results showed light allergic problems that I naturally cured.

At the end of the session, I discovered the same allergic problems in the mother as well as her daughter who was wearing dark glasses.

This was in addition to frequencies that signaled problems in the stomach and the sense of touch in her fingers.

I did not ask about her dark glasses because with teenagers, you never know if they will be offended.

The day after the treatment, the girl's mother informed me that her daughter felt really better and that her eyes were no longer red. For the past two weeks she had used eyewash several times a day to relieve the burning.

A relative's son underwent surgery on his Achilles tendon and for two months, he had had a wound that refused to heal. Using the machine, I used the inverted frequency again on the cells, in order to eliminate the aftereffects of the anesthetic and for a correct recovery of the scar left by the surgery.

After three days, the mother called telling me that the wound was now completely closed. A few days later she again confirmed the excellent and lasting results of the treatment.

The footpath is delimited on both sides by numerous mountain pines that emanate a strong curative fresh perfume, that reminded me of one of those cough syrups I had to take when I was a little child.

For a while, the left side lost itself in the stony void of the precipice below.

This is surely not a pleasant thing, walking along it at night with only the moon lighting it up: the same moon that, when I was a child, I had observed as it painted shadows on the arcade; an inaccessible mountain path with long arduous and dangerous tracts.

It was arduous and dangerous especially for someone like me, who had never had the talent for walking, least of all with my sick legs.

But I had a feeling that it would be worth it. I was constantly attracted to the figure that preceded me and it now it looked like I was filling the gap with him, as he continued to move ahead of me.

Right then, I could not recognize the profile, but my instinct told me that he would not hurt me. So I continued proudly and for the first time in my life, I started to climb the steep high mountain slope. It was then, that I remembered that I had always looked out of the window when I had stayed home with my parents.

Ever since I was a little boy I had always had one burning desire…yes, okay, it was a thing I had never even mentioned on my wish list and it was to be able to plant flags on the top of the mountains where not even plants can grow, and to see things from high up which from near seem very big.

People worry about what they have never seen; that restlessness is what it is about. I was so far above and then…a bad fall let me lose the bizarre contact with the impossible. Reality is hard and it hurts.

There are people who at sunset turn their shoulders to the setting sun in order to create big shadows.

This always left me with a sad empty sensation, perhaps because I was never a cynical person.

A terrible pain at the hip shook me: "Now the only thing missing is me not being able to move anymore.

Surely they would find me next spring." I thought so.

I started laughing, really hard; it had been a long time since I had laughed so wholeheartedly.

The strange person who was walking ahead, turned around to look at me and with his right hand gave me a signal that he wished for me to continue following him.

I stood up again, and I shrugged the dust off my hands and trousers. I bit the bullet and started walking again, battling on. I swore this time I would battle on.

Chapter XII

For the summer holidays during the hottest hours of the day, we played cards on the balcony.

That dark and shady balcony was a sort of secret shelter. There we felt at ease far away from everything and everybody.

It was as if nothing could touch us when we were there.

Other children were around as well, on top of our group.

We always knew what to do; each game at the correct time and each day had its own rhythm.

Everybody was still there. Nobody had gone away yet. There were also the parents, the smell of newly cut grass, the noise of the hammer beating the scythe, the hay sheaf carried on the shoulders of the cowhand feeding the animals, my friends Italo, Massimo and many more faces who slowly, slowly during these years lost contour and shade.

It looked as if we again had all the time in the world and we could also allow ourselves the luxury of wasting some of it.

In the following years, that passed quickly and silently like mute friends, I realized that one can't waste time. It's not like that, it was never like that, and it will never be like that again.

During the cold winters that tormented the valleys of Brescia, my play mates often invited me into the cowsheds to play. There we would keep warm and we didn't miss each other's company.

The clothes I wore were sewn at home and they were always clean and perfectly in order, so much so that a neighbor gave me the nick name "young prince".

She was always convinced that I did not go into the cowshed because I was afraid of dirtying those simple clothes but at that time my boyhood clothes were made by my clever mother's hands who sewed the clothes on me as if they were my second skin.

The truth is that I never went in to the cowshed because I could not stand the smell of those animals.

Their smell was so strong that the stench would remain on the clothes, and for many days afterwards you could still smell it on your skin; you carried it on you like a sin.

At 18:30 the local blue bus transported the workers coming back from a hard working day in the factories down in the Gardone valley.

The bus stop was right as one entered town. Children always went there and we waited for our parents in order to walk back with them along the road that divided us from our home.

One evening I happened to be late and walked as usual into the stream of the workers who were wearing their grey jackets, all looking alike. I gave my hand to my older cousin whom I mistook for my father because he had the same stature and baldness.

When I realized my mistake, I immediately dropped his hand but went on walking next to him while everyone laughed and commented on my reaction.

My interest for non traditional medicine was surely born out of necessity even if I can now definitely say that it has grown to be a passion.

For much of my life I could not raise my right arm, scratch my back or simply brush myself; these were not easy tasks.

I underwent multiple x-ray and ultrasound Scans, but no examination showed any particular problem.

One day I went together with my mother-in-law to a physiotherapist who used techniques from the Far East.

We had not made any appointment so they invited us to came back at a more convenient date.

We returned a fortnight later and during the first examination the physiotherapist pressed my shoulder and clavicle with his two thumbs.

After that first operation he invited me to raise my arm.

I raised it slowly, expecting to feel the usual strong pain but I found I could raise my limb well over my head.

This unconventional physiotherapist, in just under a minute, had completely resolved the problem that I had had for months, a problem that had taken over my mind and reduced my body movement skills.

Following this initial cure, I went to this unconventional healer on several different occasions for back problems which he regularly solved, while for my legs he told me clearly that he was unable to give any treatment.

The physiotherapist told me many times that the best thing would be to try some acupuncture, in order to optimize and obtain a result using a simple manipulation.

As my dentist and another doctor of my acquaintance had both graduated in acupuncture, I organized the opening of a studio for massages and special treatments using acupuncture.

I created a non-profit association where members could be cured at low-cost prices while being perfectly assisted by specialists.

Because of bureaucratic delays concerning the opening of a qualified studio for this special kind of treatment, I decided to close the studio and devote myself exclusively to research regarding the effectiveness of the electromagnetic bio resonance treatments.

When Federico had the psoriasis, our first holiday in the summer was always at the seaside.

Normally we went to the Marche region, but now because this illness had been cured I started thinking about a fateful cruise to north European sea.

A trip with the smell of the reindeers has always been one of my wife's wishes. Personally, to travel in the summer into the cold has never really convinced me; no sun, no sailing, no swimming, in short all the ingredients which gave me the taste of a nice respectable holiday would be missing if we made such a trip to reach Fogar.

We departed from Milan in really suffocating heat and landed in Amsterdam welcomed by a powerful storm which helped to support my theory about the real ingredients of an appropriate holiday.

At the airport of the northern capital the airport thermometer confirmed my theory indicating 15 degrees less than at Milan.

At the Norwegian harbor of Bergen a really nice sailing ship, with four masts like at the time of the 1800's, was already anchored.

We visited the city and then we started touring the Geirargerfjord.

The quantity of water that was discharged into the fiord during a period of thaw was most impressive and from every side we saw incredible waterfalls, the most beautiful one had been correctly baptized "Bridal Veil."

We arrived at the Faroe islands, that were wild, completely green isles without any trees.

The houses have grass on the roofs and sheep were everywhere.

Following a road map, I went to the post office to buy some stamps as I am a passionate collector, but unfortunately on Saturday the post office was closed.

Federico wanted to see the stadium where the Italian football team once played. Nearby, there were four football pitches where ten children were playing.

For lunch we went back to the boat and during the afternoon we saw some more life.

I asked a taxi driver if he could show us the island and he asked me if we also wanted to go to the other islands.

I thought reluctantly that my English was not good enough anymore.

With the map in my hands I insisted on a trip around the island, that was about 15 kilometers.

When we agreed upon the price for the trip, the taxi driver brought us to different panoramic views of this unusual island. We stopped to admire some Roman ruins that consisted of four stones, one on top of the other, that had nothing to do with the nice white

beaches lapped by light blue water with a fleeting view of a coral reef.

Suddenly the car stopped in front of the entrance to a tunnel. The driver explained to us that it was a submarine tunnel which connected this island with the other one.

I was amazed.

In these lost isles, where even the sheep protected themselves from the wind by hiding behind the rocks,

15 isles out of 18 were connected to each other by means of state of the art underwater road tunnels,

while we in the Trompia valley, land of one of the most prestigious firms of the peninsula, had been waiting for years for an alternative road system to substitute the present one with its overload of heavy traffic, that connected us to Brescia.

The sky was still grey as we sailed towards Iceland.

We passed the Arctic Circle and even if we still had not seen the midnight sun, it was always light and we had difficultly going to sleep.

We arrived at the north of Iceland passing along a fiord that took us to Akureyri, although without ever seeing the shores because of the never-ending thick fog that covered the land mass at this latitude.

From there, we took a taxi which took us to more waterfalls surrounded by long green expanses of pasture on which large herds of horses and cows calmly grazed.

Finally in the afternoon the fog rose and we were able to admire and wonder at the great volcanoes with their tops full of fresh snow.

The following day we arrived at Reykiavik. Finally we saw the intense blue sky again with a crystal-clear sun mirrored in the sea, the temperature having climbed to about twenty degrees.

During the home trip we exchanged some pictures with some other tourist friends. I opened a bottle of wine I had won during a game in which I had taken part while we were on board.

I noticed that one person did not drink, so I asked him: "Don't you drink?"

"I like good wine," he replied," but before I got married I ate some grilled beef and drank some good wine together with it. Afterwards I felt really sick."

I could not avoid taking a little test.

I told him to form a circle using the thumb and middle finger of his right hand and asked him to put the other hand on his stomach.

My astonished but trustful friend lost the closing force in his fingers and precisely with minimum struggle I was able to open the circle even though before it had been tightly closed.

Conserving the same position of his fingers, I asked him to put the other hand on his thigh. The power came back to him and this time I could not open or interrupt the life force circuit formed by his fingers.

I handed him a full glass of wine and asked him to make the circle again using his right hand. I checked the force with my fingers and this time they seemed so full of vigor that I took off my leather belt and put it into his hand while taking away the glass of wine.

This time the circle opened really easily.

With a simple Chinese test I could tell him that the patient under examination, himself, was beef intolerant and did not have, as he thought, an intolerance to the most ancient drink that had been loved by the Greeks, Romans, by heroes and also by the gods.

At that point his wife, who also had a puzzling allergy, asked me to check her too by using this simple test to verify the food intolerance.

I asked her to put her hand on her stomach and the circle opened. Then she put her hand on her thigh and the circle opened again very easily.

Then I suggested that she put her hand over her head and this time the circle remained closed.

I discovered that his wife has been involved in a motorbike incident; she carried around with her signs of the trauma by receiving surgical nails in one of her legs, the nails were to be taken out within a couple of months.

So I put her left hand on my watch and told her that I wanted to repeat the test. That is how I found out that she had a strong nickel allergy.

I suggested to her to look on the internet for her nearest BICOM operator who could treat her nickel allergy together with the organic residuals of the anesthetic and the operation scar which had not yet perfectly healed.

I let her know that a temporary solution would be to use plastic or silver cutlery so as to not aggravate the allergy situation.

With this simple test that can be carried out on anybody, it was very easy to get rid of the patient's allergies, something that can be repeated and effectively confirmed using the most sophisticated and suitable testing done with software for various elaborate programs for the electromagnetic bio resonance.

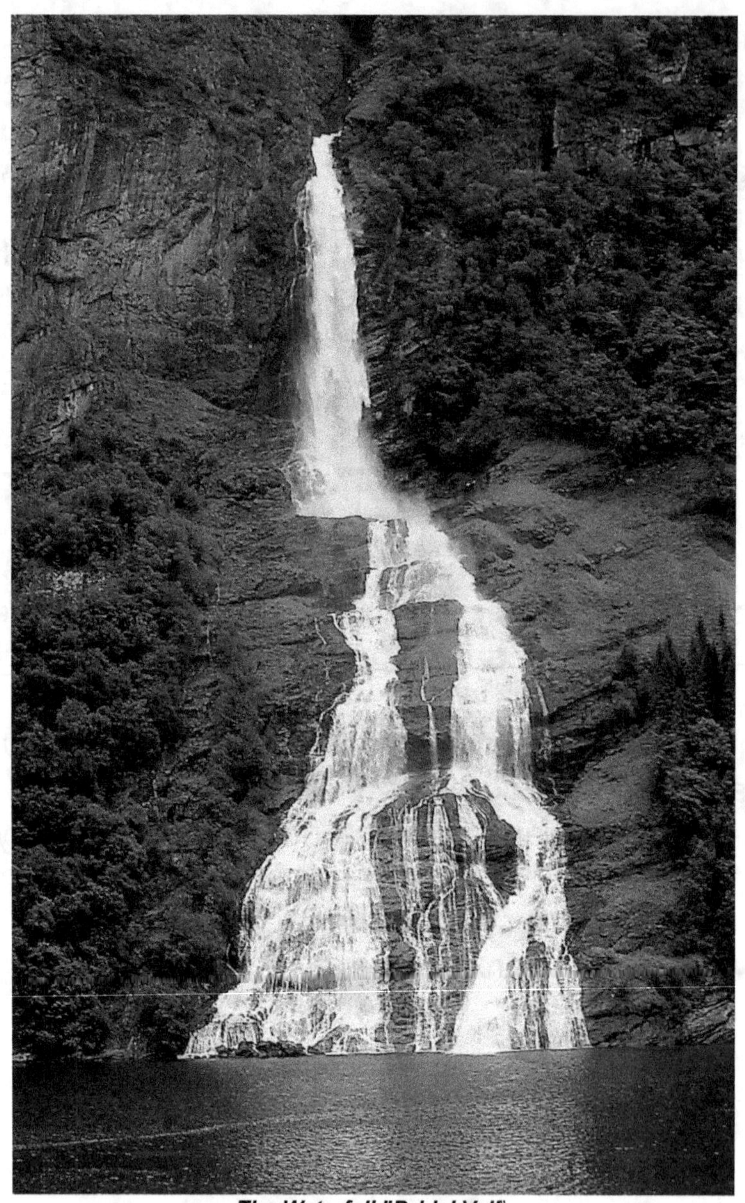

The Waterfall "Bridal Veil"

Chapter XIII

When I was a child the games I loved the most were Mechanical, such as building windmills with little metal sheets, two gears, screws, nuts and then with the help of a small handle I could move it quickly. That gave me the idea that when I grew up I would make something that could also move sideways.

At Magno, I sometimes saw my town friends and often visited the small artisan shops in the town which played a large part in the life of a small village.

Some sold guns, others weighed the metal parts, some others assembled the hunting guns starting with the raw materials.

All those small artisan shops resounded with the echo of singing that came from those primitive boxes of old and dusty radios, often hung up with a nail in the mighty stone and lime walls or sometimes placed on some solitary shelf in the middle of the wall.

The sound filled the streets and always gave a happy atmosphere; it was like living in a village of hearing impaired, if somebody had to ask something you had to remember to first turn the volume of the radio down.

One man who owned a shop in front of the main entrance to my house told me:

"Those who must work in the factories listen to different music." Then he added, "When it's hunting season I only work when it rains. I'm the owner of the shop and of my own time."

From that time on I decided to be the owner of my own time; to research that which interested me, discover what I did not know and widen my mental horizons in order to get in as much information as I could.

Living daily with more knowledge: that is what I have done in the years that followed.

My father did not like hunting. He worked in the factory and his hobby was to play cards on Saturday and Sunday afternoons in the old village tavern.

My passion for playing cards I inherited from him perhaps, even if my father had never had many occasions to play, but I often played with my mother.

She loved to play "Briscola" - definitely not an aristocratic game.

Sometimes Federico also challenged me, but afterwards he was always sad when he lost. So I always repeated to him that in life nobody lets you win, at least for me it had been like that. I don't like to lose either, and as I won a discreet amount of money at a casino, my wife took me away before I could win any more.

I love to travel by car but I have only owned cars with the usual fabric-covered seats.

Once, I drove from Brescia without interruption all the way to Cefalù, the town where I spent my sailing holidays.

Then one day my wife bought a car with leather seats.

When I traveled the first time for about 500 kilometers I felt tired and had to stop continuously; sometimes for a coffee and sometimes to refresh my reflex movements that were very difficult.

I could not understand what was happening to me perhaps I was getting old, but at my age that was not the case.

My strange beef allergy also began to affect me again as I came into contact with the leather that covered the seats of my new car.

It sounds incredible, but once I completed the treatment for the intolerances in question, I again discovered my pleasure for driving. It was common for me to drive to the seaside and back without taking a break and without any feeling of breathlessness or exhaustion.

I knew a girl who helped the nuns run the local Kindergarten. I really do not know how, but she heard about my machine and asked me if she could see it.

She was a university student in biology. I made the test on her but she did not show any particular intolerance or negativity sign concerning food. After the first meeting I spoke to her many times again, with friends, relatives and course colleagues.

I taught her the right application of the resistance test using the hands. She wanted to know much more from me, in particular she wanted explanations regarding the use of phials, frequency and the use of the rudimentary travel Birek that I lent her several times.

She also wanted to see as many notes as possible regarding patients with specific symptoms. In particular, she was interested in the treatment I gave to people with Parkinson's disease because in fact she was writing her degree about this terrible and degenerating illness.

After her degree she decided to become a cloistered nun but before she went in to the convent she took her parents to see me for a treatment.

The father did not have peace because of his daughter's decision while her mother was more resigned.

A few months later I received a phone call from a nice, kindly voice who asked me, "Do you remember me?" On my mobile phone was written: biologist.

"Yes of course, but I thought you had taken your vows to enter the convent?"

I asked her.

"I am still here and we are allowed to call for special emergencies. I have used the Birek on a fellow nun.

She has no food intolerance but I think she has allergy problems and as we cannot leave the convent I would like to ask you if you could come here with your machine," she replied.

"With pleasure", I replied," but I do not know where you are and when I can visit you."

"I will pass you Mother Superior and she will give you all the information you need."

As soon as I had received the right information I quickly loaded my tools and I was sitting in my car.

Beside me was my wife, looking quite curious about this new adventure and wary of the trip we had to make to see what life behind the walls of the cloistered nuns was like.

The stereo system played a CD that made us more attentive. It is always difficult to understand why in certain moments some simple notes associated with a good text can give us the feeling of strange and irrepressible passions; our eyes become wet and the emotion becomes bigger and gives way to strong emotions.

The words of the song that was playing said' "We know where we are born, but we don't know where we will die."

The thought crossed my mind. I would have liked to have stopped the car, get out and speak with Mirella, telling her… in the distance was the convent silhouetted against the hills. It seemed suspended between earth and sky or at least this is what I thought I could see.

I had never been in an enclosed convent but my wife had, so she helped me wheel the trolley with the electromagnetic bio resonance machine. In front of us was a small waiting room delimited by a grating in ironwork.

This was the only place from where we could speak with the nuns.

I needed a chair for me and a chair for the patient. So I went over to the door that separated the visitors and went in a sitting room where there was a cheap-looking table with four chairs of similar quality.

In the presence of Mother Superior, who did not once take her eyes off me, I completed the tests on the nun who had needed my help. I found out that she had a pollen and dust mite allergy. I found out that she had a pollen and mite allergy and with the set of five elements I also found a malfunctioning of the kidneys, of the stomach and of her entire metabolism; all associated with a moderate debilitation due to depression.

During the treatment the biologist also came and spoke a bit with my wife. Mother Superior was amazed that from these results I could find all the organic incompatibilities. With a severe voice she asked if I also had time to visit another sister.

She introduced me to a nun who came from South America. The machine immediately informed me that she had problems with her stomach and general metabolism but no allergy.

I also started the treatment on her. Then I tested Mother Superior and the biologist and applied the correct frequency on both of them. I used the power treatment that the German professor I had met called "optimism treatment".

Then came the moment to use the Birek. The biologist took her leave from us saying that she would like to hold onto the Birek that I had lent her just a little bit longer. She thanked me for my willingness to help them and said, looking deep into my eyes, that she would pray for me.

During the trip back home I asked my wife: "As you can also speak with stones, what were your impressions?"

Her answer was immediate, but soft with a bit of emotion: "To tell you the truth, I felt a bit uneasy. However, in that silent environment, I found total serenity in the biologist and even if she looked so pale she was very beautiful."

For me, it was difficult to understand how such a nice, young, intelligent girl could leave the world with so many human inventions, emotions, irrationalities and pleasures for a wish to repudiate herself completely.

Her own life continued behind the walls of an enclosed convent where she could bring with her only objects of primary necessity and of little value. However, she had chosen among her few possessions to bring the Birek that I had lent her, a frequency signal tracer which had been refused by universities and hospitals.

After more than one year, while I was writing this book, I was not surprised to receive a phone call from the Mother Superior of the enclosed convent who, with an enthusiastic voice gave me the communication that all the patients under treatment had received great benefit. She asked me moreover, if I could came back once again with the bio resonance machine for a nun who had skin problems and who could not be cured using traditional medicine.

My answer was…yes.

My father in-law had never had much trust in my machine although he frequently suffered during the night from leg cramps. After the correct treatment for tendons and ligaments he did not have any more problems.

Mirella and I often had differing opinions; for example I like go to one dentist and she to another.

One day her dentist proposed a little operation called "crown extension" which she decided to have.

After having this operation I could still see her suffering caused by strong gum pains several days later.

It was then that I decided to make the correct treatment for her.

The day afterwards she felt a bit better.

For a minor issue, she had to undertake another operation. This was exactly one month after the first operation but the usual treatment for the scar was not necessary anymore.

Several times I have tried to involve doctors and specialists of different branches of traditional medicine in order to inform them about the successful results obtained by using the body frequency stabilizing machine.

Once, I telephoned some dermatologists telling them that my son had been completely cured from a severe psoriasis illness by using the electromagnetic bio resonance. But their answer was always negative and sometimes completely disinterested.

Calling some professors by phone is surely not a good way of leaving one's card. So through a friend

who was a bank executive at the hospital in Brescia I got an appointment with the head of a hospital allergy department.

I presented myself at his office in the department and tried to explain the German machine to him. I informed him that this machine was immediately able to test for allergies and that the test was not invasive.

It was also in my interest to verify the good functioning of the machine and I had 400 phials which I put at his disposal free of charge for two afternoons a week when I could go to the hospital or the outpatient clinics to make the tests.

He dismissed my argument within a few minutes telling me to consider that I was speaking with him in a public structure and that he was not permitted to use tools without the approval of the Department of Health and that even if I gave him the machine as a present he would never use it.

As I was leaving he called me back and told me that if I were interested I could speak with the assistant who was the owner of a prestige private practice.

I waited for some minutes, while the young female doctor was inoculating some curative products in the arm of a patient.

When she had finished I repeated the same things which I had already explained to her superior and tried to give her my mobile number.

The answer was curt and distant. "Give me nothing.

Call my practice. You will find the number in the telephone directory. My secretary will give you an appointment."

I did not see any need for continuing our discussion so I left.

Sometime later a boy with allergy problems came to me.

He had been at the hospital and the doctors had examined him. He brought the test results with him.

My tests confirmed most of the analysis results.

On the paper of the hospital tests was the name of the doctor responsible for the analysis and I was surprised to find that it was in fact the dean of the university of medicine.

Again I contacted my friend who worked at the bank and he organized an appointment for me at the university.

I went there with the Birek, the phials of the main BICOM test and with the chemical analysis laboratory report for which the dean had been responsible.

The professor anticipated my discourse by saying that he did not have much time for me.

gave him the documents I had in my hands and said to him: "This is the report from your laboratory. I did the same test using this tool and the results corresponded." I asked him to lay his arm along the desk in order to make some tests without touching him physically.

The dean complied and stretched out his hand, so I used the Birek.

After a bit I told him: "In one minute I have given you a complete checkup.

Your organs are working well, you do not have any food intolerances, you do not have any lung allergies but I can see a presence of palladium.

This is a heavy metal and the machine is able to eliminate it. I have noticed the presence of this metal in people who suffer from a genetic illness such as Parkinson's disease."

"But I am feeling perfectly okay!"

The angry professor answered me in a stentorian voice providing an index of good health.

He regained his composure and a with calm voice said, "In the university we do less experiments but it could be that your tools would be of interest in the analysis department. Would you like to speak with my assistant?"

Hopeful I went back to the hospital where I made the same test on a lady doctor. I discovered she had both a beef and palladium intolerance.

"As I am vegetarian it is not a problem for me and also, if my superior is not interested in your machine, why should I be?" the young lady answered me ironically.

However, the test results left a nagging doubt in my mind – if I had found palladium in both doctors, how many other medics among doctors and nurses could be affected by this kind of heavy metal?

I have not seen or heard any more from that famous doctor so I hope he is still feeling well.

While a person of whatever sex and age is watching television during the cold winter evenings, if he puts both hands upon his navel he can move heat within his whole body frame. In five minutes he can beat the cold.

Who can tell if the professor knows it?

The top of the mountain seems nearer. Looking through the valley I can see the built-up areas becoming smaller and smaller, receding into the distance.

Now I can see the person who is walking in front of me. I can distinguish his features. His face shows a strong and determined character. The skin of his face being partly lit by the setting sun has taken on a rosy red appearance.

Only a few meters are left and the strange character has already arrived on the flat top of the mountain.

I observe him carefully while he places some small stones which he has quickly collected to form a ring.

In the middle of the ring he puts some small shrubs and dry sticks. It reminds me of some rite as he then methodically starts a fire.

I observed the smoke which spiraled like a tornado into the sky, while a singsong melody floated softly into the air.

The repetitive sound was being composed of a few vocals put into a strange melody and all this came towards me. It looked to me as if it wanted to get inside my intestines.

A strange reaction and a glad sensation of warmth overcame my body.

As I walked faster, breathing seemed completely normally. I did not pant anymore and the echo of my breath was not thundering in my ears.

My legs were strangely light. I did not feel my hips hurting anymore and my pelvis seemed in harmony with the movements imposed by my legs and other body parts which were suffering from the climb.

He was sitting down crossing his legs and with rhythmical movements began to whirl the flat part of his right hand towards the sky.

He put the flat part of his left hand at the height of his stomach and pressed lightly down on his solar plexus.

I have known that one's hand can be used as a frequency revelator.

The span is a door; it is like a reader who sends messages to the mind. It is the sixth sense to all intents and purposes.

I have always thought that one's hands are the intelligent part of the human body. I have often seen them move for strange reasons, for example to make a gesture, to protect against harm, to stroke, to touch during the dark when we are looking for something placed on the bedside table in our bedroom.

But now it was the first time that I was seeing this movement.

I continued observing him with an almost pathological attention while with the same hand movements

penetrating the thick smoke which rose from the improvised fire, he brought the smoke screen nearer to his body. Then his hand moved from the bottom to the top of his face, attracting towards himself big clouds of smoke.

It looked as if he was smoking a cigar but his mouth was closed.

I was only a few steps away from him but I could not take my eyes off him and watched him with avidity.

The melody, which was impressively repetitive was still coming out of his diaphragm.

It was as if he were hypnotizing somebody, but there was only himself and nobody else.

Chapter XIV

I The faded portrait has sat for years over the fireplace of my new house. It has been painted in clear lines showing her young and sympathetic. In all this time she has never aged.

Her look is always the same, even during winter evenings when it rains outside and the window panes offer nothing better than a misty vision.

He left a few years ago. With a gun in his hand, he followed some thief who during the night had entered his manorial villa.

I noticed him immediately. He looked like an old hero coming from a frayed cinematographic history of town, his beard and moustache bringing boldness to his face

that was not only marked by deep expressive wrinkles but was in harmonious sympathy with his long grey hair that rested on his shoulders.

He had been introduced to me as the new person responsible for the branch where I had worked for a while, but if I have to be sincere, his appearance was a bit retro, so I immediately imagined it to be that of a cowboy of bygone times and thus my impression of him remained.

That painting that was a portrait of my wife had been painted by him. It was his personal

present when I got married.

For sure, such an acute person with a strong sense of intellect and duty could scarcely conceal his strong artistic vein, even when sitting behind such an important desk.

I observed him at work and often smiled as I thought of his kind "killer" methods but it wasn't that big a mistake to imagine him in a western comic book, because that was in fact how he left this world and even when I think about it now, it is impossible for me to remain serious.

Then I become sad for a while, and I feel that sense of anguish again when I think about Chiara's story.

At first when I still wasn't capable to use the electromagnetic wave machine for human treatment, I limited myself to only carrying out diagnostic tests, marking the food intolerances and in the meantime suggesting the correct personalized diet.

By eliminating foods that brought negativity to the body I began to understand how I could obtain good results by using the machine and this was not only for Federico's psoriasis: I also found significant healing methods for headaches, backbone pains and symptomatic treatments in cases of obesity.

A convivial banquet is surely not the ideal place to explain about the importance of avoiding noxious food but when invited with the insistent understanding that I explain myself concerning this argument, I could not refuse to clearly outline that the absence of specific substances was a really good treatment against organism complications.

That evening during a discussion I found an unexpected ally in the form of a university professor, who, in support of my theories, told those curious and skeptical people present about the eccentric events that had happened to his astronomer colleague who had organized an expedition on the Himalaya to observe the stars.

The colleague in question had been tormented for several months by a strong pain in his back but had refused to give up his trip, as it had been the dream of a lifetime.

Without any particular problem, he had obtained all the necessary complicated permits for a successful trip, the departure being exciting even if he was worried about his health.

The usual acclimatization with base camp was over 5.000 meters and in this case there wasn't much of a chance to find a great variety of food.

In a village without commodities he could only get sheep's milk and sheep's cheese, that were his only means of support for two weeks, but amazingly during this period of time, the annoyingly persistent pain in his backbone had gone completely.

It was now six months since his return and because he had continued to eat just and only products derived from sheep's milk, his backbone pain had completely disappeared.

Chiara had come to me exactly during the first month of pregnancy but I did not carry out any test on her because as it was written in the BICOM users and instruction handbook, the use of electromagnetic waves on women in the first months of pregnancy should be avoided.

She came again during her third month unable to believe that the machine had shown a double intolerance against beef and wheat for her.

Chiara is the daughter of a near relative of mine and in my list of genetic studies concerning the Sabatti hereditary traits, the results of her tests had shown that she had never had a wheat intolerance. This in itself was very normal for the inhabitants of the Trompia valley where only a few people showed a light wheat intolerance.

For a correct understanding of the research tables concerning my relatives I also did a check on her husband who came from Sicily and found he was wheat and almond intolerant.

During the first month of pregnancy Chiara told me that after each meal she suffered from a gastric illness. She had therefore been advised to eliminate exclusively bread, pasta and beef and since then she had felt much better.

A fortnight after the birth of her child I remembered to check the new mother again, and this time she showed only one intolerance, for beef, while the wheat intolerance had disappeared.

But her baby daughter showed just one intolerance and that was for wheat, just like her father.

Chiara thanked me for her alimentary diet which had resolved all her problems and for the fact that I had committed myself to the health of her newborn child many months prior to her birth.

She would be glad if I could also act as godfather for the child.

Doubts about everything regarding the course of my life, as always, reared their ugly head. Had Chiara's husband in all probability, passed his wheat intolerance to his newborn child, who had then transposed it to the organism of the pregnant woman?

What were the phases that generated this complicated transduction mechanism? The genetic re-establishment was still not clear for me but ever since, I have seriously started researching this problem, often testing women at different stages of their pregnancy and in association with these results, I started carrying out tests on their whole family units, their partners and sons included.

Approximately for half the cases tested, the results underlined a double food intolerance: one of the two corresponded to what we found in the adult male, while children only had one intolerance, either from the mother or from the father.

For the women who were evidently far gone with their pregnancy I used the Chinese test, inviting them to repeat it again at home using all the food products they had and to use less make-up because up until now, I could for example find no eye pencil that had not shown to be bad.

Using the results from the Birek I compiled a list of foods that had to be avoided for their own health and for their future baby.

I got another confirmation from a boy who had gone on to get a degree in physical therapy. He had experienced an anaphylactic shock by eating nuts. I took the ring test using some of this dried fruit and he was amazed that the intolerance had taken away a great deal of his energy. I did the treatment with inverted waves and immediately afterwards he did not experience any more negative reactions.

I asked his parents to come and visit me, so that I could test them.

The father showed the same intolerance as his son, while the mother was only pollen allergic.

The woman told me that during her pregnancy she had often eaten dried fruit but during her last month she had often thrown up because of her upset stomach.

I also have the same negative intolerances as my son; I do not like kiwi, so I avoid it.

On the other hand Mirella used kiwi for regulating her digestion during her first uneventful pregnancy.

However, during her second pregnancy with Federico that same fruit did not have the desired effect and she often had to go to hospital, the doctors failing to connect her illness to something she had eaten.

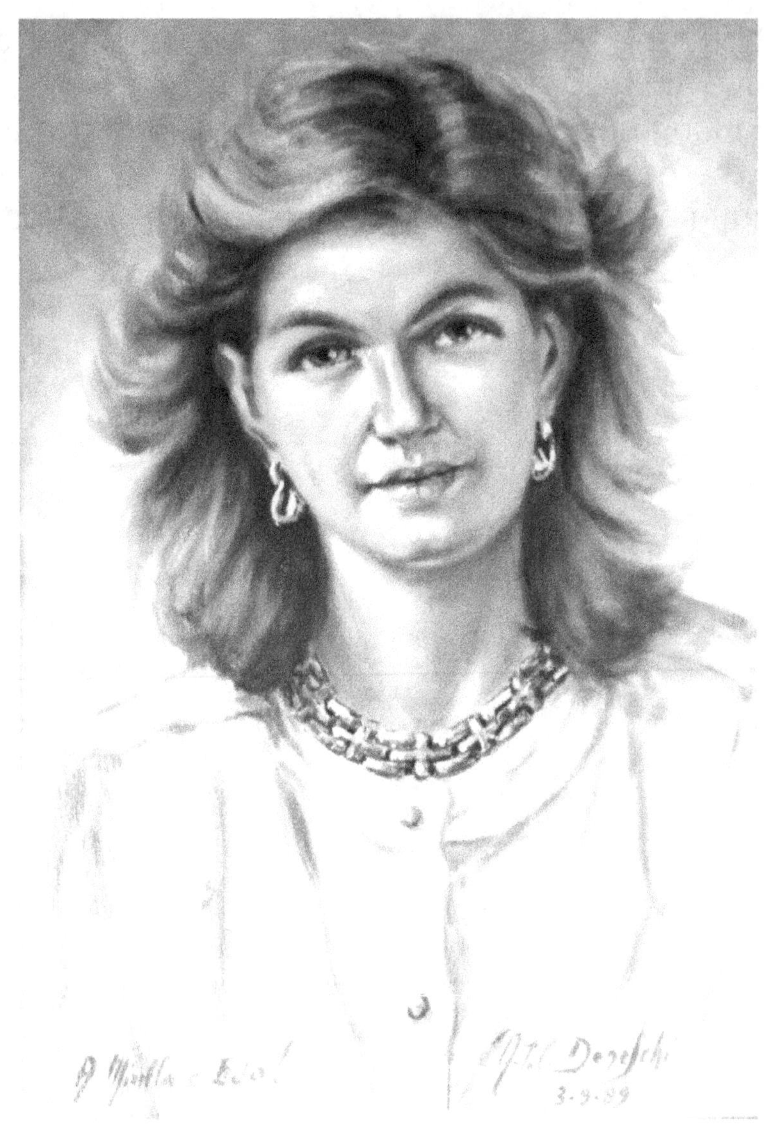

Chapter XV

I am near, so near as to be able to hear his breath.

The smoke keeps on rising and expanding into the sky.

The dirge fills every part of my being. I am calm, very calm. Perhaps I have never been so calm.

I realize that the continuous melodic repetition of the same sentence, in I don't know what language, is the psychosomatic preparation for an extraordinary event, an event in which I must I must face without any particular emotion, agitation, fright or frustration.

The sort of concentration that I am feeling at this precise moment is of a very high conscious level.

I am feeling that I can remember or memorize every space/time event.

For a brief moment I detach my gaze from my mysterious mountain companion and I look toward the valley.

Evening has already come at the foot of the hill and the houses are already in darkness.

The streetlamps have been switched on, illuminating the roads swarming with white, yellow and orange lights creating a sort of B shape, or so it seems.

I feel surreally distant, I know that I am experiencing something fascinating and mysterious but my fixed point of reason tells me that I am here.

The man who is sitting next to the fire is real, the smell of smoke from the burnt twigs is real, the harmonious voice that reaches my spirit is real and the big hawk that continues to fearlessly circle above of us is real.

The wind that often accompanies sunsets at this height is also real, as it shakes the leaves of the curious trees that seem to whisper among themselves.

I would like to speak, ask something but his hand sign tells me not to.

Now the hand on the side of his heart moves the smoke and it is as if he is spreading it on a vertical cloth that is invisible to me.

Contours and shades of his clothing mix with the smoke screen that continues to grow thick as it encircles us.

I look around me but I do not see anything because grey-white smoke is completely surrounding us in a kind of embrace.

It is like being in a cinema looking at the flat screen in front of you and then imagining that the same screen starts entwining itself into a cylindrical form, inside which you stand, and you see scenes from the film at 360° all around you.

I remain silent but I do not hide a feeling of contemptuous embarrassment, the only form of emotion I feel, that eventually disappears.

Now the tone of his voice lowers, and it seems as if his singsong has saturated the cylinder of smoke that wraps us.

My heart jumps with a jolt, bringing me back to reality;

I feel the taste of adrenaline when on the impromptu screen, human figures start appearing.

Men and women, big and small, who pass incessantly onto the film of smoke.

I can recognize some of them, old friends from when I was a teenager, people of the town where I have perhaps spent the best times of my life.

I can clearly distinguish some faces of the people I have treated during all these years of continuous research.

They pass near me, disappearing to leave place for new figures that begin to compose the

multitude continuously forming in the central part of the fire, where the twigs are burning unconcerned with a crackling noise.

I observe the scene in between disbelief and disorientation but I am not afraid. Being here is what makes me calm and I experience no fear.

Many faces that I know well, pass in front of me.

Some of these have been people to whom I have given suggestions concerning their body harmony, such as people whom I have checked simply for pure scientific knowledge. There were also women and girls whom I have helped at particular moments of their lives. I took care of their more serious, persistent and seemingly unsolvable problems or simply helped them feel more beautiful, healing persistent skin blemishes of various kinds on their faces.

What continues to escape me is the form of thought that the man now sitting with crossed legs and folded arms, is trying to convey.

I think I hear a murmur but I cannot distinguish the words.

There seems to be no sense to what I am hearing as the sentences are confusing, with tones sometimes overlapping, like in a theater during the break when there is incomprehensible chatter.

At this point I think I need to approach him if I want to listen clearly to what he is whispering.

I have to sit down just as we usually do at the theater when whoever is sitting nearby speaks and hears the various topics perfectly, but whoever is standing or is far away only hears the confusion of voices that seem completely senseless.

I move nearer to my strange new friend. I sit close to him and try as much as my inherited difficulty will allow to cross my legs, copying the position he is already in.

I now hear clearly what he is telling me and it is the silence here that I feel. I am fully aware of the silence,

like when you are sitting alone on a church bench during a sultry summer day.

The silence of your thoughts sometimes can make a deafening sound.

I remember now a sentence that I read in an ancient manuscript that was recovered from a church in Baltimore :

"Pass quietly between noise and haste and realize the peace of silence."

And then more: "Stay at peace with yourself, with others and with God, however you conceive him."

For a long time I had forgotten that I had read that ancient parchment but now, here, in the most absolute silence, I remember every single word perfectly, as if I had composed it.

Silence fills up the void we have inside us. I have never been so silent since the day I was born.

I don't feel the need to speak anymore, I am not distressed by having to ask verbally about anything, it's enough for me to feel well, so well like I've never felt before.

To feel well in silence, to observe myself in a way I never have before.

The need to know takes us away from the Supreme, and knowledge makes our thoughts noble.

Knowledge comes from silence, from knowing Ourselves, from letting our spirit speak.

The melody I heard before was his soul singing.

In silence every soul can sing.

He is saying all these things without speaking and every notion he proposes, passes silently before me.

Now I know what pushed me to search continuously.

The figures disappear and the smoke disperses little by little into the air. I look at my digital watch that I always wear on my wrist like a real timekeeper. I smile as the hour, minute and seconds all show the number eight.

Eight like the rotated infinite, like the trajectories of mountain hawks, like…

I know I've been lucky not to miss the appointment that everyone of us has with their own being.

We do not often realize that we have only this one unrepeatable occasion to get to know our own wisdom, as we are so often engaged in listening to the noise.

Now I know that everything I ever looked for served the purpose of getting to this point.

I knew those I had examined up until now, those with whom I made my therapeutic tests, often with success sometimes unsuccessfully, I knew those who passed me by in all the years of my life, I felt like I could do something more for them but I never found out what it was that I could really do.
I knew everybody else, all of them: their faces, their worries, their physical problems, their alimentary habits and even their allergies, but I did not actually know them, just like I didn't actually know myself.
Yet it was simple, it was enough to climb this low hill and meet with this strange Indio, while the smoke encircled us. It was enough to watch a hawk wheeling high above our heads and seeing the number eight from another angle. It was enough.... it was enough to observe silence.

Chapter XVI

The potential of the BICOM electromagnetic-wave machine is incredible.

I believe that the scarce diffusion of this important instrument has been caused exclusively by the elevated cost of purchase.

When the sale representation, at one time exclusive, was also publicly awarded to NES MEDICA in Milan I noticed a price reduction in the machines and phials of over 40%.

With the new tariffs, this type of equipment surely would become more approachable for first-time operators.

The courses in Milan started to be held by Italian teachers and operators. Among these I found, as speaker for food intolerances, Daniele Zamparelli from Pescara.

We had already met during previous seminars, and it was during these we had exchanged opinions about our experiences, agreeing about taking the opportunity to write a book on our daily treatment experiences.

When I went to the sea side in the Marche region for a few days of summer relaxation, there were multiple chances to carry out the kinesiology test, to detect allergic problems both on Italian and foreign tourists alike, as well as on the staff of the hotel I stayed at.

If I detected any serious or urgent cases I directed the patients to Pescara where Daniele directed the Metab Srl, a center of homeopathic medicine that relied completely on the bio resonance machine.

Decidedly younger than me, after completing his Ph.D he had attended specialization courses both in Germany and in Switzerland, on top of collaborating on numerous studies and at medical group practices as diverse as dentistry, fitness centers and plastic surgery in Rome, Bologna, Chioggia (VE), Sora (FR), Aquila and Oristano.

Our experiences were decidedly different. I occupied my time noticeably with the Sabatti family problems, therefore with the hereditary aspect, in a limited context, with people belonging to numerous family groups that had high percentages of specific alimentary intolerances that I cured in a few therapeutic sittings.

He, on the other hand, had a vast territory with specialized problems needing numerous consecutive sittings but limited to one component of a family.

The occasions to see Daniele in person again as opposed to just speaking to him by phone were few and far between and it was on one of these rare occasions and precisely during the presentation of the new and adjourned BICOM version, that we were both surprised to see each other and equally satisfied to learn about what

the innovative high-technology equipment could do.

Something of great interest and not only for those using the machine, was that the new frequency updating also envisaged the exit of low modulations between 1 and 10 hertz.

The new frequencies made the absorption of waves on part of the body easier, and thus eliminated the long and sometimes superfluous "unblocking" therapies that allowed the patient to be more receptive to the following therapeutic emissions.

What was even more sensational was the greater number of programs, both for testing and healing,

that did not need to be supported by the phials, because many of the already known frequencies both for metals and environment allergies were directly inserted in the machine during the programming phase, thanks to the greater know-how acquired by the BICOM producers.

This makes specific adjustments of the phial products unnecessary, as it enough to update the previously inserted frequencies by loading them onto an external drive.

On top of this, the maintenance costs regarding the deterioration and expiration dates of the phials were avoided.

At this point my peremptory observation was, "... It's science fiction where we are now! ". Daniele's immediate response set me straight:" We were already living in science

fiction. Now we've moved on."

We were both completely aware of the fact that these tools were used more for the causes of allergic onset than for the effect that the allergy symptomatically caused.

The electromagnetic waves were surely able to improve the sporting performances of athletes, freeing them from unconscious presences in their organism of all sorts of toxins, free radicals, excess of lactic acids and all that, and providing them with clean organic energy from elements found in the environment.

One of my nephews competed in pro bicycle races, in the younger athlete category, and he had an iron deficiency according to blood tests. The team doctor prescribed some tablets but after a fortnight of uninterrupted use, the test results were the same.

The doctor insisted he should continue to take the tablets, and that produced no satisfactory results.

The boy, who was notably worried, came to me desperate to resolve this urgent problem.

With the Birek I noticed a negative effect in the prescribed tablets. I then moved on to the BICOM machine putting a tablet at the entrance and testing the medicine as if it were an allergy product. The program with inverted waves allowed me to perform the therapy on my nephew, giving a frequency time of about three minutes.

Once I had finished the therapy, I again performed the test with the Birek; the result was clearly positive.

Following the treatment, blood tests on the boy were so good that my nephew's doctor told him that the new values for iron in his blood were very good, and that he might even have been wrongly tested.

Another young cyclist complained of constant calf pain.

From the test I noticed acute problems at his tendons and ligaments. Consequently I carried out the support treatment that lasted several minutes.

The following week he placed well in race standings, and then won two races. He told his team mates that since he had held the spheres in his hand with the electromagnetic frequency contact of that strange machine, he had never suffered anymore cramps or pains in his legs.

During the winter training of the younger cyclists and junior teams, they authorized me to perform some allergy tests.

In these tests I noticed that 20% had alimentary intolerances and pollen allergies, 10% had exclusively alimentary intolerances, while 15% had exclusively pollen allergies. In the team were also two athletes from Eastern Europe who did not have any such problems.

All those who suffered from pollen allergies confirmed that they had problems in spring during the flowering time and that they felt better later in the season.

Within a short time I made a survey of all allergies straight in the locker rooms, showing that these tests had been carried out without chemical organic alterations to the athletes and that all tests were completely not invasive.

An amateur runner asked me if I could check his banana intolerance.

The kinesiology test did not show any kind of energy

Decrease, while the Birek moved vertically, a clear sign of positive effect. I thus told him that he had no banana intolerance and that the fruit in question is greatly favorable for him.

After a pause, the young man respectfully explained that he trained five hours a day but often after two hours he suffered from cramps.

Since the time his sport doctor told him to eat a banana a day he did not experience this trouble anymore.

Every month he came to Brescia for a checkup, and Inquired on my availability for a BICOM test.

He phoned me one September evening and after a few minutes I found him in my study.

I began the 5 elements check-up. Everything was all right; no signs of allergy.

At that point, I went through the complete range of therapeutic stabilizing programs, finally finding a blockage in the lower back region.

I therefore performed the computerized therapy suitable for his problem.

The frequency therapy was finished within five minutes.

While I was informing the young man about the therapy, he told me that it was when he ran downhill that he had the most problems.

He also informed me that the Poli, the winner of the New York marathon who came from Brescia, was organizing the Italian participation in the following NY marathon.

The race would start at the beginning of November and he told me that he would have loved to participate. He knew that he did not have much possibility of obtaining a good placement, but he was convinced that to participate in this competition would anyway be a great experience.

I therefore recommended he visited me a few days before his departure in order to perform a test and a possible preparatory therapy. I asked him moreover, to let me know keep me updated on his back problems after the therapy.

A fortnight later an elderly gentleman phoned me introducing himself as the young man's uncle, the runner who had visited me. He informed me of the good results his nephew had experienced from my work and could he also make an appointment with me.

The elderly gentleman had an intolerance to beef, allergy problems because of some pollen varieties and the set of the five elements also signaled some problems in his liver as well as his spine.

Also on him I performed the usual electromagnetic waves therapy.

In the last week of October the young man called me to have his final check-up prior to his departure for New York and his participation in the most famous marathon in the world.

The set of the five elements showed an acute inflammation of his tendons and ligaments. Staring at him squarely in the eyes I asked him, "Are you sure you want to run this marathon? My machine isn't showing me comforting signals."

He quickly answered in the affirmative, almost as if he wanted to disguise his state of internal worry but the tone of his voice was not lying.

"To tell you the truth," he told me," I have been completely resting for a few days. I'm undergoing quite a lot of massage treatment but the real problem is, I have already paid for the competition's registration fee and for the flight ticket."

I performed the appropriate therapy for the various underlined problems, but nevertheless I was not convinced I'd obtain a good result. I recommended, that whatever happened, when he came back in Italy, he needed to come see me.

I remember that time I followed the marathon with particular interest. It was won by an African athlete, trained by a sport doctor from Brescia.

The following day, after the competition, I read with great satisfaction on the internet that our athlete had finished the marathon in three hours and two minutes.

He had run the second part of the competition faster than the first part, reaching the eight hundredth place out of forty thousand participants who had completed the race.

A week later he called me, telling me enthusiastically that he had run a good race without too much effort and that he had exceeded his personal record with that result.

Moreover, he kindly asked me if I could meet his physiotherapist who was very interested in aspects of body frequency through electromagnetism.

At that point I understood that the result had been very important and probably completely unexpected for his team manager.

I met the runner again in the mountains two years later. This time he was preparing himself for the Berlin marathon, informing me that the preceding year he had again participated in the New York race but this time it had been rather disappointing.

Contrary to the first marathon for which he had undergone therapy with my machine, the second time he had gone to New York his finishing time was worse by over twenty minutes.

He asked my availability for a visit and a possible energizing therapy using the BICOM.

Four days before the Berlin marathon I carried out the treatment for his tendons, ligaments and inflamed muscles.

On Sunday evening I was curious to see the race standings on the internet. I discovered he had obtained the six hundredth place out of forty thousand participants, also reducing his time to about five minutes under three hours; exactly thirty minutes less than for the entire American race.

That was surely an excellent time and great position, considering the attitude and the potentiality of the athlete in question.

I was really satisfied, personally not having done a great deal of work but I remember well how it seemed as if I had also raced.

After returning from Germany, however, the sportsman was less satisfied. "I ran the last kilometers much slower in comparison to the position I had in the first part of the competition," he told me.

As we had agreed, I completed the therapy for his rehabilitation, re-equilibrating muscles, tendons and ligaments.

I thought he had taken a break for some months, but, on the contrary, two weeks after Berlin the young man participated in a half marathon and the following two Sundays in hill running.

In all these three competitions he had always overcome his personal record.

When I saw him again I reproached him spontaneously, "I made the rehabilitation therapy for you to recuperate and not for you to exert yourself in competitions!"

Excusing himself with low tone he answered: "I felt myself to be in full form; the muscles did not hurt me and I had a great time overtaking the other athletes who had a much better personal track record.

However, the other participants had not been envious.

Rather, someone even asked me if I had changed my training method. For this year the season has finished, but next year, with your help, I am sure that my preparation will certainly be the best."

I could not blame him. This runner had given me much greater satisfaction in comparison to other athletes, completely involving me in his own enthusiastic way.

The point of the stone arrow was turned to the East.

Laying on my heavy study table, it was looking at me.

It pointed to something, maybe the direction of the rising sun, the light and... Lucio: yes, he gave it to me.

As if it were a strange amulet with unusual powers he had placed it into my hands.

Certainly Lucio has walked down many roads, not like our marathon athlete, but in a different way: yes, in a completely different way.

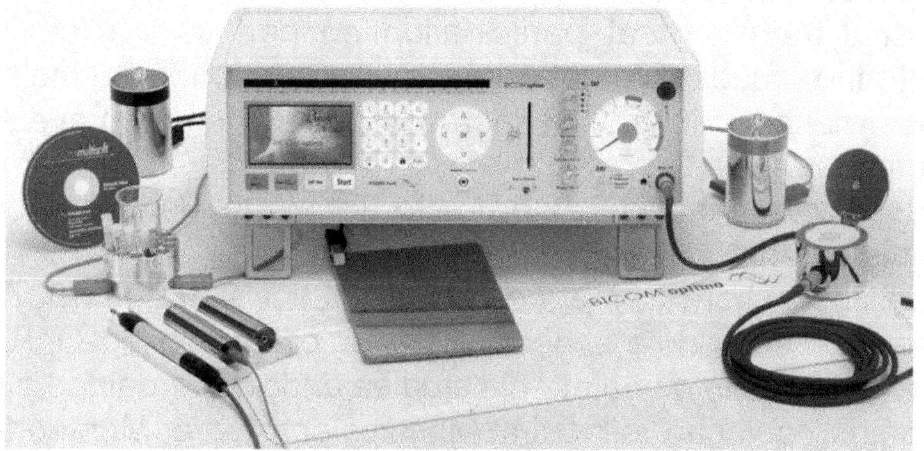

BICOM OPTIMA

Chapter XVII

I did not how long it takes to get to Patagonia in Argentina for men.

Not how long or how much time it would take to get there, but by what mysterious ways we could get there.

It was a different kind of funeral I was attending today.

As usual there's great participation on part of the inhabitants of Magno to the procession that brings a village member to the cemetery, and I hear neither cries nor desperation but only some prayers and low murmuring.

We are accompanying Father Lucio Sabatti to his last place of rest, next to his parents.

He had been born in Magno on Saint Lucy's day in 1937 and like me, had finished middle school at the Salesiani College in Chiari but then had gone on to complete his studies and was ordained a priest.

My mother took part to his first Mass celebrated at Monteortone near Padua in 1964, of which I still have the photograph.

There was nothing in particular to notice. The village people, including my mother, were all dressed in their best clothes.

She was the "prima donna" standing on the right-hand side in the first row, to the left of the father. She had thought so much and for so long about this exciting trip to take part in one of the events that had caused much commotion and betting in the village.

To be chief female mourner was an important position and even if it was only for a Mass, she would not have missed it for anything.

Lucio had come a long way: yes, a really long way. On the border between the known world and the Antarctica ices, where rocks become luscious vegetation and where centenary Patagonian conifers rule.

When I was a little boy I liked to play with a bow and arrow and often had more than one occasion to build one myself.

For the long thin stems I used hazelnut, which could be easily bent into the correct arc shape and was readily available in the woods that surrounded the village. For the arrow shafts we used thin metal sticks that extended the cloth of broken umbrellas.

But, arrows with points of stone I had never seen before, or at least not of that kind, rudimentary, made from black raw silica lava or from quartz stone, clear, almost transparent and extremely fragile.

Every five years, Lucio came back from Argentina for a short period of rest and human closeness to his friends and relatives.

When I worked at the bank, in charge of currency exchange, I often had to convert Italian lira into dollars.

Lucio, with a beaming smile on his face, complimented me on the favorable exchange rate which, rounded off with my mother's donations, became a congruous and conspicuous amount.

In exchange for the money he usually gave me some stone arrow heads, hand made by Trelew Indio, to use on the tips of my arrow shafts.

These men still live today by hunting the guanaco as their main survival means.

As a sign of great honor and deep tribal memory towards the cult of the dead, these atavistic points, scarcely of any value in the west, are the only talisman that accompany the deceased on their last trip into oblivion towards the valley of the dead.

Ten years ago speaking about the economic situation in which Argentina was struggling, I was surprised that father Lucio approved the government decision not to return loans that had been given by financial structures and world credit banking systems.

In his opinion the crisis was so great and had become such an enormous burden for each Argentinian citizen, that the people could not survive any further taxes.

A few months earlier, I visited him at his parents' house, a few days after his arrival. He had not lost the beautiful habit of smiling lavishly before answering, although I noticed when talking he had great difficulty in using our language, as he was barely able to remember the words. However, the words he could remember the best were at first in his village dialect, then came Italian.

The Argentinian economic situation was still very serious and he disapproved of the President's dissolute behavior, wasting a lot of public money on several changes of outfits during the day and on continuous palace parties.

When he visited us a month before his departure, his main worry and absolute priority was as always, the poor people of Trelew in Patagonia, where he would have liked to be buried.

But his tired and worn-out heart had kept him here with us, in the small sunny village cemetery, forever.

Using the internet, snooping here and there on various sites, I found a eulogy edited by an informative magazine called, "Newspaper of the Patagonia."

These were the precise words that had been written: "Lucio died in his village, where his family have great respect and care for their dead and from where the Sabatti family originates.

The people loved him. They held him in great respect and the help he received for his work often came from that place."

Lucio laid in the intensive care unit of the local hospital during the last days of his life, but the doctors were unable to help him.

Others suffering from a similar problem often manage to overcome the crisis and return to lead normal lives.

The church, that during normal Sunday functions and festive occasions usually has more than necessary capacity, today was so full that people were everywhere. Seats in every corner were occupied and benches even had to be brought out into the open, so that everyone could attend Father Lucio's burial.

I decided to stay by the right-hand altar of the Romanic church of cruciform construction, as from there I could easily follow the coffin. My thoughts overflowed, moving so quickly I could hardly control them and it wasn't without difficulty that I was able to contain the emotion climbing to my throat.

The voices of the readers and the liturgical songs sounded as if they came from far away. Then, when for moment I come back to reality, I understand that people singing are covering the notes of the organ.

It was as if everybody wanted to participate, testifying with their voices that they were there, that they were there to accompany a man who had travelled so far with his feet and had left so many imprints in the hearts of each one of us.

Right here and now, while I am thinking about Lucio's funeral, I am oddly serene. It is with great satisfaction and quiet voice that I am able to repeat to myself, that I... I was there on that day.

Football (for Americans, soccer) was the most practiced sport at Magno.

A few years after the war, our parents had built a football pitch for six-player teams.

On the hillside starting with the ground work, rigorously done by hand, they had dug some terraces for the public, similar to an archaic Roman theater.

The stones that they had found were used for filling the containing walls, thus obtaining the appropriately flat area where the new and loudly applauded parish sports field was born.

Time as usual worked against our human efforts for the village stadium. The fragile protection nets were now destroyed, and there was a deep groove in the central part of the ground dividing the pitch into two parts and making it impracticable and unusable to promote the purpose for which so much effort had been wasted.

It was now our turn to restore the work that our fathers had started, by modernizing the crumbling structure with new, effective locker rooms, thus allowing the local football team to participate in the provincial tournaments called C.S.I.

To collect funds, various initiatives took place, from lotteries to fund raising events. My job as happened many other times in my life, was to be the secretary or cashier.

Alfredo got very busy with that French accented "rrrr" of his – the result of his few teeth – and he kept the morale high in our happy and hard-working group.

We still laughed years later about his great wisecracks.

As I'm here alone, thinking about things that do not make me laugh at all, I well remember his most famous wisecrack: "experrrts."

As I placed the pen on the table, I had another look at the photo of us on the sports field. Almost as a premonition in that photo of us you are absent and I think, "Alfredo, you were great, you were really great."

You, Alfredo, had correctly made the extremely difficult forecast of the World Championship finalists in Spain. You correctly guessed not only the outcome, but the two finalists as well, a combination that was deemed impossible by sport journalists and television speakers who followed that prophetic Spanish event.

You were the first one to leave us, the fault of a tumor which brought you to the top of the hill, to the peak and then even further; up to the sky.

A boy, following a fall in the mountains, had been hospitalized in intensive care.

I had spoken to one of his relations concerning the post operational effects of the anesthetic on the human organism. I explained that my machine could pick up

the signal of the presence of such toxins many years afterwards. Following that conversation, she invited me to visit the patient at their house, where I went with all the equipment.

The worried mother told me that her child complained a lot for about pain in his right arm.

The orthopedics insist in saying that the forearm fracture was completely set and therefore he should not have cause for so much pain.

At this point the parents did not exclude new surgery, even if they personally held an opposing opinion.

I use the spheres, usually correct only for children's therapy. I completed the first treatment to cauterize the anesthetic while for the remaining part, I carried out the pollen therapy using inverted waves.

A sixty year old man from the village, after feeling unwell in his car, had been brought to the intensive care unit, where he remained for about ten days. After a couple of months at the hospital he returned home.

I visited him at home. He often complained about dizziness, and his stiff right hand which was so rigid that it was a complete impossibility for him to open it.

With a rejected voice he told me he had always been a draftsman but now he could not hold a pencil in his hand, not even to write a simple note.

In this case as well I took my machine to his house.

The task proved difficult for me on this occasion, because he could not hold the small spheres that were needed to transmit the impulses to his semi-invalid right hand.

I treated the anesthetic and his allergies to grass and dust mites. Following that, I carried out a treatment to reactivate the functions of his liver and articulations, recommending that he help himself by drinking a lot of water.

A few days later I received a written note from him, " With thanks from your Juventino friend."

The weak candle light flickers on the side of the wall where the great hearth sends shades that give a sense of warmth and company.

Certainly, I knew a lot of people.

But today I don't want to think anymore, I don't want to feel my stomach stringing with tomorrow's thoughts anymore.

A sentence I read somewhere said that for every day there are enough worries.

I still have Lucio's smile in my mind. I blow out the candle and rake the last remains of the fire. I look around me and it's as if I'm not alone in the room.

I turn and see an amulet, or at least I have always thought of it as such: a small seashell from our eastern sea coast.

Memories from when I was a child and I went to the beach come back to me; the most famous seaside resort at that time was Cesenatico.

I loved to hear the noise of the waves, but what attracted my attention more were the shells that laid on the beach: I walked along looking at them with interest, but without touching them.

They were inanimate, but they did not give any sense of being dead to me.

And that is exactly how I felt earlier today as I looked at Lucio's coffin. It was as if he were still here.

Rather, now that I think of it, that sense of parochial unity lets me think that perhaps he has never gone away from Magno.

This strange small village seems to never release its children, either in life or in death. Certainly, people often forget, the village never does!

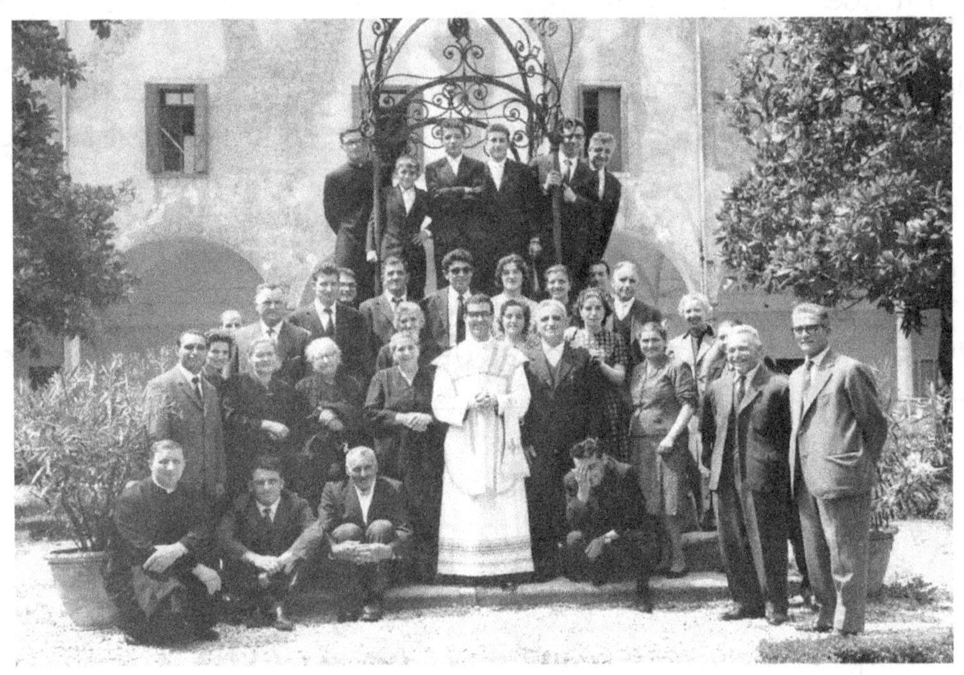

Monteortone a. D. Lucio's first Mass

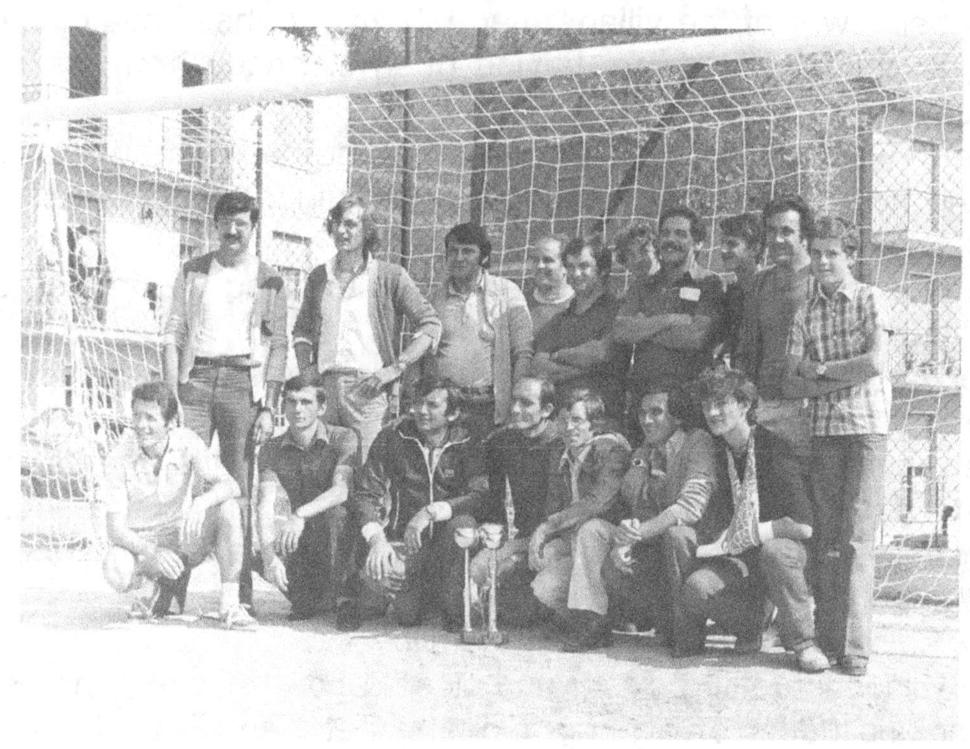

Standing on the left Edoardo nice memories, nice friends

Chapter XVIII

The bell tower of the village made its mighty bells heard. From the peak the sound was clean, having been cleansed from the noise of everyday life.

When I was a little boy this sound was the prelude to the adventure of being able to go out during winter evenings when it was already dark.

The just occasion was when we went to evening Vespers or to serve at Holy Mass.

Afterwards, we used to meet in the old streets of the village to play chase or to ring the door bells on houses.

Then, between laughter and shouts along the little streets and narrow paths of the village, we would meet up again at the end, in the small square in the center of the village to tell each other about how, where and when...

Now I am slowly walking down the hill.

The village is getting closer and closer and I have the impression of smelling the odors of evening dinners that I smelled when I was a child.

Some smells stay with you forever.

On the coat of arms of Magno are, under a weapon in the form of a shield, four stone towers that defend an eagle situated in the center:

These represent the four founding families of the village population.

The native families that gave origin to the entire population of Magno are:

The Sabattis, who were known, according to the ancient popular motto, for Science,

The Tanfoglios who were known by this primitive definition, for Knowledge

The Rizzinis who were the eccentric and unpredictable branch of the village community, in fact with a fanciful term in dialect, they were maliciously defined "the unbalanced,"

and finally the Zolis, the dominating ones.

Rinaldo belonged to this last family and over the years had collected much information regarding the families of Magno. It was him who gave me my paternal genealogical tree.

It started from 1630 and analyzed genealogy up until 1900; from then onwards I was able to complete it myself.

This was a work of enormous talent, paired with historical research, taken to great depths and at my express wish, after some weeks, he was also able to give me information concerning one of my maternal family branches.

I developed such a deep interest for this research, that I started to look among the old parish registers for the information belonging to other genealogical trees, those of my grandmothers, one Sabatti and the other Rizzini.

All four family trees which I found confirmed in the Book of Souls dated 1680, that for over three hundred years, my ancestors had never moved from Magno.

Now that I was in full possession of my roots and finally had dates and names of those who belonged to my family over the centuries, I was able to read, or rather scrutinize, this information every time I felt the need for it.

I heard the noise of a fly that maybe irritated by my presence or maybe attracted by the smell of my body, came threateningly close to me.

I immediately recalled my passion, as a kid, for catching flies to give to the "ciuina", which is the dialect term for the minuscule black and white bird that I kept for years in a cage in the window of my father's house.

I had always taken a very good care of that vivacious insect-eating bird, and despite applying a lot of effort and passion, it still took many years to train the bird completely.

I only succeeded in conquering its trust when I fed it with flies for its meals. When I sat at the table, it was a spontaneous reaction for me to grab them with a quick hand movement.

I react automatically when I see a fly, it is a spontaneous gesture for me. Grabbing flies while they were flying around amazed Federico, and he always observed me with great interest.

Sometimes he gives it a try, but as it is always hopeless he persists in cheering me on.

Good result consists in catching them from the front, while they are scared and fly slowly in the opposite direction towards danger.

I have always pondered deeply about life and death.

Now in my mind I see the small cemetery appear, where I have accompanied some of the people I have loved most in this life.

I try to think not only of relatives but of friends as well, but my mind right now refuses to remember them.

Today has already been sufficiently intense and perhaps by a primitive form of defense I now prefer to not remember any longer.

It is certainly true that children often know what to say without any Aristotelian pretensions of great knowledge.

A few years ago, while I and Federico were together visiting the graves of our ancestors, with an uneasy feeling, he suddenly pronounced a sentence that has buried and rooted itself inside my memory:

"Dad, after a long life I would like to be buried here.

In this place where the sun always shines we are also nearer to the sky."

Personally, I have never pondered this matter.

Even though deeply attached to my origins I have always thought that when the adventure of this world ends, I would like to live in other spaces and in other times, therefore to be buried here or elsewhere is not an integral part of my being.

A contradiction appears in my thought: Lucio, who loved his country and his earthly mission, was sure that in Argentina he would have been useful both when dead and when alive.

We people of the village, perhaps for a sort of slight egoism, too, have buried him in our small country cemetery, although we know well that his heart remains even in death divided between his Indio people and us. We are perfectly conscious that he was ours. We have shared him. Now he is of both worlds.

I, just like him, know that my roots are and always will remain well-planted in this place, but I also know that I do not belong exclusively to Magno.

With soft footsteps I continue my descent, and I see the rectangle of the sports field appear.

During winter evenings when I look at old photographs again, I see myself as I was then, thin and with a very out-of-date dark moustache.

I was ... we were very young, but as I pull the photo near me, it's like I can still hear their voices.

I have never forgotten the vocal tone of any of them and I feel their whispers are still inside me, despite the years that have quickly passed by, taking me down other paths.

It is strange how the first imprint of knowledge remains unchanged through time.

I surely have never forgotten my old friends, not even those who decided to depart for other seas or better, not even those who have left these seas.

As a child I often went into the village square to play or to call my father for supper during the long summer evenings, when even the sun never seemed to want to go to sleep.

I now go near and start looking around me.

The colors, the houses, the windows and even the moldings of the eaves are still the same, in this place where time seems to stand still.

I see my father again, looking at me shaking his head while he lights up a cigarette. Well, I don't see him again, it's as if I'm seeing him again.

However it is all still the same, everything is the damn same.

Trees and flowers, smells and objects, noise and fluttering sounds, everything is as it was, as it has always been and perhaps will be forever.

The village square, the meeting place for long endless talks, where we waited for our friends to decide what to do, where the children waited to decide what to play, where everybody waited. In the piazza, we waited for everything. We also waited for things that never happened.

I have arrived at the place where I parked my car.

I turn the collar of my coat, sit down and while knocking my shoes one against the other so as to remove any residues of mud still attached to the soles, I give the slope one last look.

The anger that was inside me has faded away.

I am oddly at peace. As always, only when I return to this place is my mind granted a sense of peace.

While driving down the tortuous road into valley,

I roll the car window down a bit to allow a healthy gust of good fresh mountain air to enter.

That air, sometimes terrible, that could sting my face during winter nights, when I got up to peer into the village road from the entrance of my father's house.

This trip, or better this segment of the trip that I have now crossed, has given me a definite internal certainty.

I now know for sure that everything is made to be discovered and used in the best possible way.

Just like I know that everything that exists in Nature, even if we do not recognize its true and intrinsic properties at a certain moment, carries the solution for every illness.

Just as in the law of opposites there is right and wrong, light and dark, hate and love, everything and nothing,

I also know that for every known or unknown illness, nature has already prepared her precious antidote.

But our knowledge progresses by degrees.

Over the centuries we have been romantic, illuminated, learned, foolish, but never sufficiently able to understand all about the universe that surrounds us.

My research in the field of bio magnetic properties, has convinced me that everything, every molecule and every atom of which each object is composed, radiates external waves. It would be sufficient to have the correct knowledge to read the right modulations, to have intrinsic knowledge about the correct frequencies and give the correct impulse to every bad constructive form that dominates us, and they could perhaps be defeated...

Arriving at home I found a new patient in my study room.

He had arrived a little earlier than his appointment time.

He expressed great curiosity about my work and wanted to know the way I performed treatments on people.

He had been plagued by skin problems for many years.

For several months, the palms of his hands, with constant regularity, had been filled with multiple small, painful cuts.

This problem had forced him to make many and at times useless specialist appointments, in the most disparate hospitals of the Italian peninsula.

While I was preparing the equipment, he started to tell me that he had decided to come to me upon suggestion from a dear friend.

His friend had spoken to him about this strange machine that used no invasive tests.

I completed the general test, that immediately underlined a serious environmental problem.

I therefore directed the tests and my attention to the set that produced the diagnosis.

Texting phial after phial I finally discovered the incriminating element: Hexachlorobenzene.

Personally I had never heard of this word and did not even know what it was.

Immediately I sat in front of the computer, wrote the incomprehensible word and was surprised to receive an answer from the internet so quickly.

Hexachlorobenzene: chemical element used in pesticides and parasitic sprays, provokes occupational illnesses, affecting the hands in particular, and it is the principal cause of this kind of dermatitis.

I was also amazed about the way my equipment for electromagnetic bio resonance had found the allergy that had instigated this annoying coetaneous degeneration.

Considering that in Nature hundreds of elements exist, besides compositions and solvents in various chemical combinations that could have been the real cause of the problem, the result from the software that integrated the equipment came in a very short amount of time.

In a couple of minutes the exact reading of the frequency modulation was formulated, so as to carry out the right treatment.

With traditional medicine, this would have required various appointments and for the patient, hours of invasive allergic tests with the risk of the illness worsening during the research phase.

I also decided to carry out the simple kinesiology test on the patient.

With great amazement, he realized that he was losing a large part of the force in his finger.

I invited him to support his hands on the armchair rests and placed the two brass spheres on his palms.

With inverted waves of the modulation analysis I completed the treatment, that lasted five minutes.

At the end I carried out the manual test, but I was unable to break the circle formed by the fingers of his hand. Which meant the treatment was successful.

After having recommended that he drink lots of water in order to facilitate the disposal of the residual toxins in his body organism, I said goodbye to him with the express requirement of getting feedback on the treatment result and the dermatological development as soon as possible.

An ancient motto of the Native Americans says: "A leaf that falls makes more noise than a forest that grows."

In the case of my new and unusual patient, just like with so many of those who have received benefits from the treatments that I completed, I never received any more updates or news.

It is quite the opposite when I casually meet people in the street.

For instance: the mayor of the village where I live, confirmed that ever since his allergy has been eliminated, he has always felt well. And the sportsman I treated several times points with his finger to his head where his hair is growing, ever since he eliminated milk from his diet.

Then there is a client in the bank who introduced me to others as his personal doctor, as well as the healer of his blemished skin.

Ever since I was a child, in order to overcome nervousness, I would switch the old table lamp on and off, while staring the wall.

This simple gesture was as if I wanted to connect and disconnect my mind like a command to my thoughts, getting rid of the anguish that often took on exaggerate proportions in my little boy's mind.

I turn around and look at the cabinet where a vast collection of metals and quartzes is showcased, placed with care onto the glass shelves, in order to allow the lamps to illuminate them with the correct intensity.

Every single stone has its own peculiar story and has been placed there at a specific moment in my life.

As I approach, unconsciously and frantically I start to press the switch.

I stop, my mouth stretched in a broad grin.

This time, I do not have white walls, nor do I need to stare at something. I can see what I have put away and what my path caused me to store, like a fleeting but intense testimony of a period of my life.

The metals constantly change color as they reflect the light, while the quartzes allow the brightness to pass through, changing from shade to shade, from blue to yellow until they become pink.

It is as if this explosion of colors calms my mind.

I want to change the position of the stones.

With the correct refractions, I am certain that I would succeed in getting a harmonious symphony of colors, but I also know perfectly well that this fanciful operation would require a lot of time.

So I think to myself, "One of these days I will certainly do it, yes, perhaps I will do it tomorrow ... yes I will do it tomorrow.

And then again another day, another time and another season after that."

Besides searching, we ought to learn to acquire knowledge and experience from everybody.

Now I know ... you try.

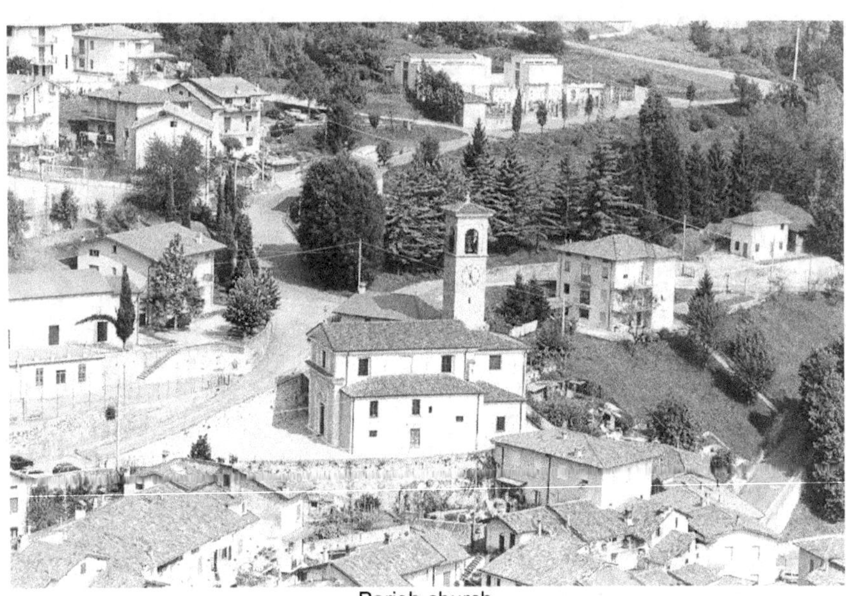
Parish church

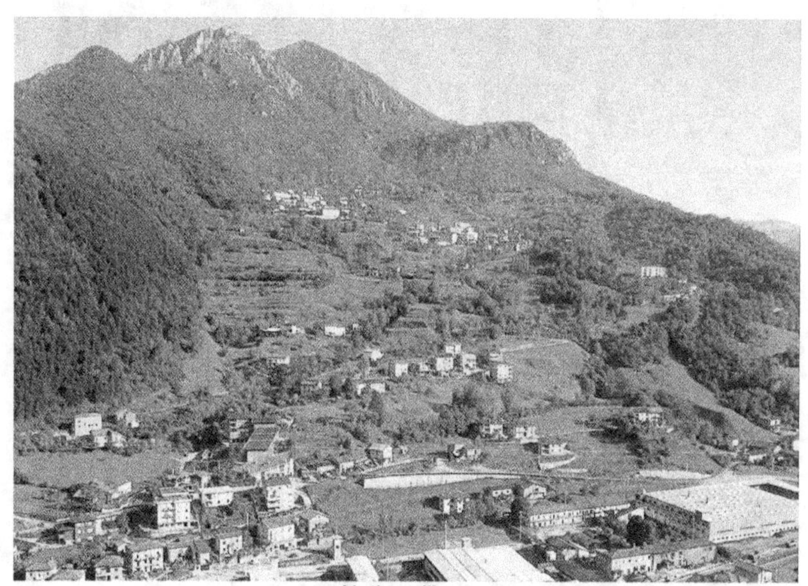

Native village

ANTENATI PAPA'

SABATTI	SABATTI
maria	1596 PIETRO
1630 CRISTINO	1628 GIO MARIA
maria	maria
1660 COMINO	1660 CRISTINO
catta	angela
1703 GIOEATTA	1710 GIO PIETRO
pasqua	margherita
1741 GIUSEPPE	1751 BORTOLOMEO
vittoria	maria
1780 GIAN BATTA MARTINO	1790 LUIGI
domenica lechi	maddalena sabatti
1815 CARLO	1815 BORTOLO
domenica sabatti	pellegrini francesca
1859 GIOVANNI BATTISTA	1845 MARTINO LUIGI
imelda sabatti	zoli cecilia
1884 CARLO PIETRO 1944	1884 FRANCESCA SABATTI 1916

1913 LUIGI MARTINO SABATTI 1968
caterina tanfoglio

1951 EDOARDO SABATTI
mirella lucchini

1990 LUCA SABATTI   1993 FEDERICO SABATTI

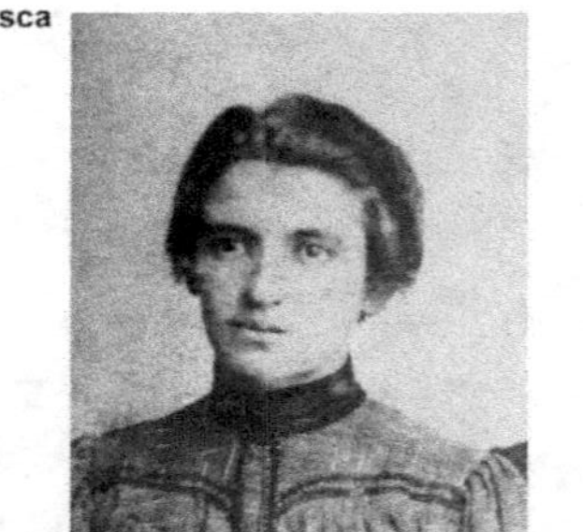

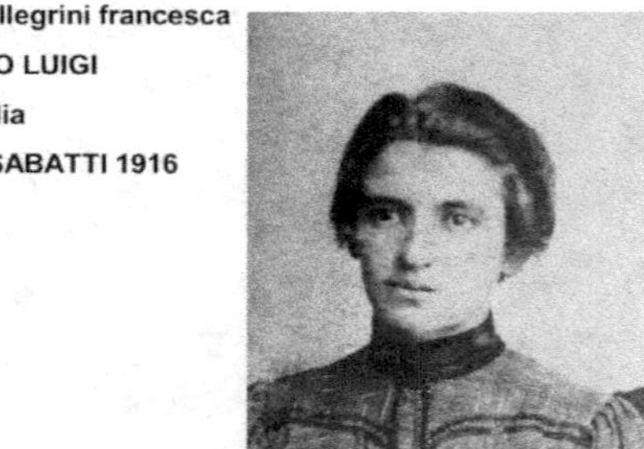

ANTENATI MAMMA

TANFOGLIO

1540 ANTONIO TANFOLLIO

1570 YOVITA TANFOLLIO
maddalena carli
1598 ANTONIO TANFOGLIO
margarita
1643 GIOVITA
catta
1683 ANTONIO
maria
1730 MARTINO MAFFEO
maddalena
1763 GIUSEPPE GIOVITA
catarina sabatti
1813 GIANNI MARTINO
aurelia pellegrini
1838 GIUSEPPE
caterina sabatti
1887 ABELE GIUSEPPE

RIZZINI

1613 LORENZO RIZINO
1643 GIO MARCO RIZINO
afra
1673 STEFANO RIZINO
margarita
1715 GIAN MARCO
lucrezia
1752 GIAN MARIA
maria maddalena
1775 GIUSEPPE MARTINO
catterina contessi
1808 LORENZO
giulia giovannelli
1860 FRANCESCO
marta bertuzzi
1898 ROSA RIZZINI

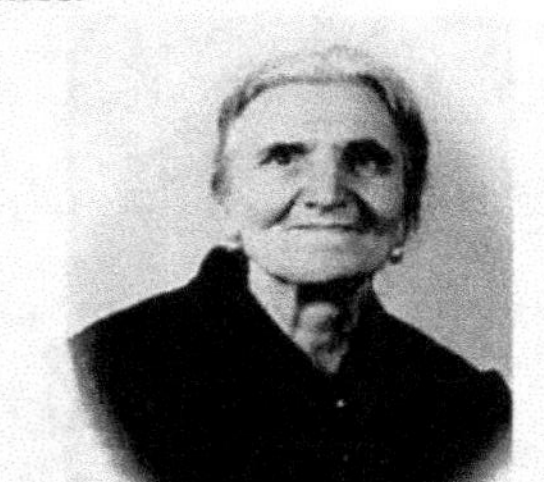

CATERINA TANFOGLIO   Palmira Tanfoglio   Marta Tanfoglio   Franco Tanfoglio   Assunta Tanfoglio

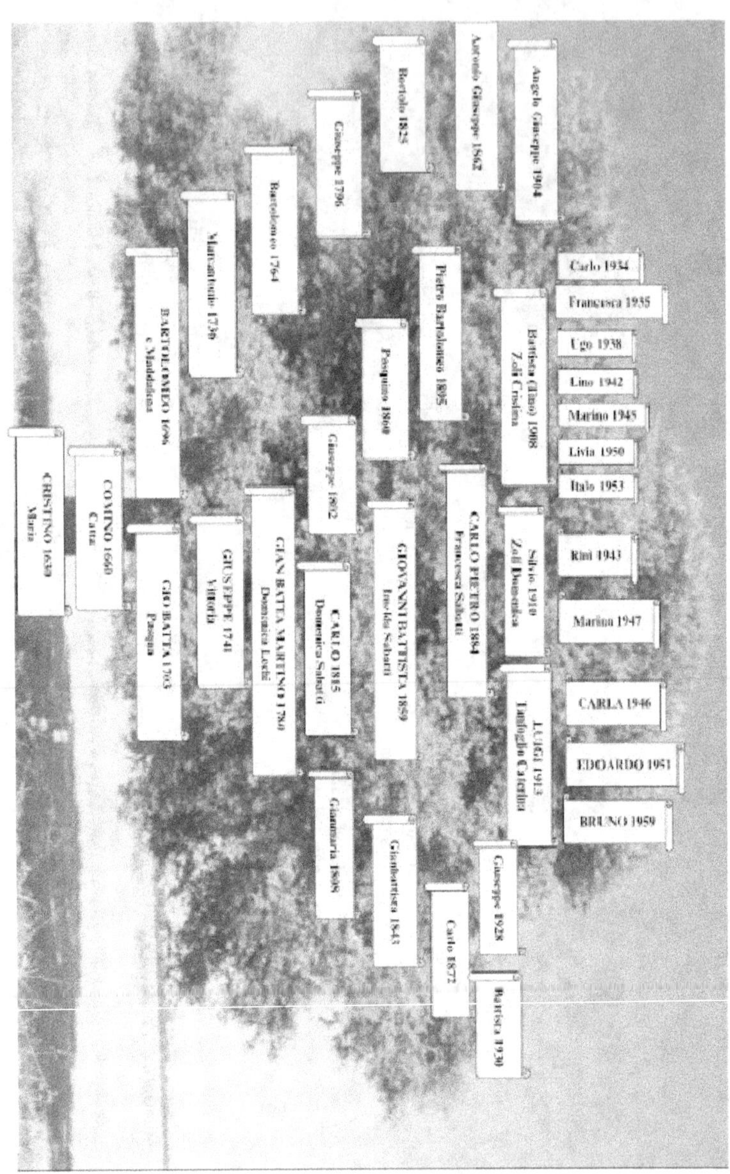

1680 soul book.. Families of my ancestors

Sabatti Comino

Rizino Gio Marco

Sabatti Gio Maria e Cristino

Tanfoglio Giovita

INDEX

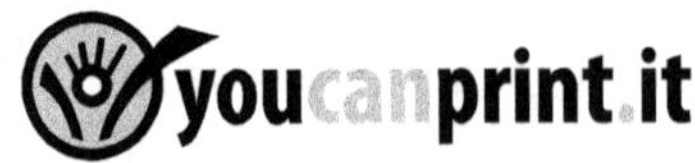

Finito di stampare nel mese di Settembre 2017
per conto di Youcanprint *Self-Publishing*